HYPOTHERMIA

HYPOTHERMIA

CLINICAL ASPECTS
OF BODY COOLING

Analysis of Dangers
Directions of Modern Treatment

Edited by
Sylweriusz Kosiński · Tomasz Darocha
Jerzy Sadowski · Rafał Drwiła

Translated by
Andrzej Górka

Jagiellonian University Press

Cover design and poster by
Jan Stanisław Baran

Publication was supported by Krajowy Naukowy Ośrodek Wiodący

Publication was supported by
the Faculty of Medicine
of Jagiellonian University Medical College
(Leading National Research Centre 2012-2017).

ISBN 978-83-233-4063-8
ISBN 978-83-233-9377-1 (e-book)

www.wuj.pl

Jagiellonian University Press
Editorial Offices: Michałowskiego St. 9/2, 31-126 Cracow
Phone: +48 12 663 23 82, Fax + 48 12 663 23 83
Distribution Phone: +48 12 631 01 97, Fax +48 12 631 01 98
Cell Phone: +48 506 006 674, e-mail: sprzedaz@wuj.pl
Bank: PEKAO SA, IBAN PL 80 1240 4722 1111 0000 4856 3325

Contents

Introduction

In every hypothermia care it is important to have a good organised chain to enhance survival for the patient. In hypothermia accidents chain starts with the first responder knowing the algorithm – No one should be declared dead before being warm and dead.

This mantra should be spoken out by everyone in the hypothermic chain all the way to hospital. And if someone in the chain is a non believer, the other persons around must rise there voices and say – "the three other golden rules of hypothermia Never give up, never give up, never give up" because these approaches saves lives.

As victim of hypothermia caught under an ice in a frozen gully for 80 minutes in 1999 I am a living example of how well it can go for a patient if the responders do not give up.

After about 2 hours and 45 minutes with CPR I arrived with helicopter at the University Hospital of North Norway in Trom; and was rewarmed on ECMO from 13.7 degrees.

I know there are other patients saved from just as low temperatures and knowing they may be alive because my story has been told over and over again makes me happy.

That I was a trained doctor when I had the accident and now are able to travel around and tell my story to health personell give meaning to my life.

I would like all hypothermic victims to get the same chance as I did.

Reading this book is a good start organise your hypothermic chain.

Anna Bågenholm MD,
University Hospital of North Norway

1

Hypothermia as a Disorder

Sylweriusz Kosiński

Department of Anaesthesiology and Intensive Care, Pulmonary Hospital
Tatra Mountain Rescue Service, Zakopane, Poland
"Heat for Life" Foundation, Cracow, Poland

Incidence and causes

Effects of cold onto human organism have been described already in the antiquity but hypothermia as a disorder was recognised only in mid--twentieth century [1]. According to the official sources in the United States hypothermia causes 1,500 deaths yearly, in Poland 300 to 600 deaths are reported *per annum*. Unfortunately, the exact data concerning incidence and fatality rate are not known. Many cases of hypothermia remain undiagnosed on account of a simple fact: almost all patients have their blood pressure, heart and respiratory rates measured, in many, pain intensity is also evaluated, but temperature measurement is not a part of routine practice. Incidence of clinically important hypothermia (excluding traumatic hypothermia cases) among patients admitted to emergency wards in Poland is estimated to be 5–6 cases per 100,000 citizens per year [2].

Although hypothermia is commonly understood to be characteristic of cold climates, it is worth noting that it can develop any place on Earth any time of year. It is beyond doubt that cold environment and major heat loss are factors most predisposing to hypothermia. If the impact of low temperature is significant and properly functioning body heat retention mechanisms fail, we speak of primary hypothermia. Hypothermia however er can develop as a secondary condition accompanying other disabilities and homeostasis impairments deteriorating thermal regulation [3, 4]. In both cases the underlying principle is a simple disproportion between heat generation and heat loss.

Thermoregulation

Human organism is homeothermic, i.e. it possesses the ability to maintain stable core temperature regardless of external conditions. In fact, homeothermy undergoes more profound and more precise autonomic regulation than circulatory homeostasis. In certain circumstances, when defensive mechanisms of the organism fail, heat loss becomes superior to heat generation and body temperature decreases. At this moment a cascade of organs and systems dysfunctions occurs, leading to death unless therapy is commenced.

Human organism disperses heat by means of three processes: conduction, convection, radiation, and evaporation. In various conditions each of these processes can have different share in global heat loss [5–7]:

A. Conduction is a process of heat transfer between bodies of different temperature remaining in direct contact. Because volume of heat loss is directly proportionate to the area of contact, this mechanism is of special importance in cases of water immersion.
B. Convection is a process of movement of air heated on body surface. The faster the air movement, the greater the heat loss. In practice, the major factor influencing the rate of convection is wind force. It is believed that this heat loss process is of greatest importance in moderate and cold climates. Importantly, proper insulation may entirely stop this heat loss process [5].
C. Radiation is a process of energy transfer by means of electromagnetic radiation emitted as a result of motion of particles. The greater the difference between body temperature and temperature of environment, the greater the heat loss. Because of this, radiation becomes most significant heat loss process in environment colder than −30°C [5]. Unfortunately, elimination of this heat loss mode is practically impossible, regardless of thickness and type of body cover. It is worth

remembering that infrared radiation can also be absorbed, thus sun, fire or other strong radiation sources can provide heat gains.

D. Evaporation is a process of transferral of heat to water particles which causes a change of state of matter. The process is the basic mechanism of cooling in high temperature environment. Interestingly, it can be of major importance as a heat loss mechanism in people wearing thick and waterproof clothing (e.g. firefighters). It is also worth noting that about 10% of total heat loss occurs via airways – mainly due to evaporation.

Human organism has been equipped by evolution with exceptionally efficient mechanisms of maintaining normothermia. Thermoregulation centre in hypothalamus controls both heat production in metabolic processes as well as its dissipation. The most important role of thermoregulation centre is maintaing constant temperature of internal organs (core). The remaining, peripheral parts of the body (shell), change their temperature depending on circumstances and serve as a buffer for heat dissipation as well as accumulation. This goal can be achieved by means of specialised, thermoregulatory arteriovenous anastomoses located in skin of peripheral body parts, which can accept up to 10% of cardiac output in broad ranges of flow [6, 7]. In cold environment anastomoses constrict, skin temperature drops, and heat dissipation is halted. As hypothermia aggravates, resulting shock promotes global vasoconstriction of microcirculation, which further limits heat loss. If thermal deficit continues, mechanisms of heat generation are initiated. Shivering begins after temperature drops by about 1ºC below the threshold for closure of anastomoses. Shivers occur in synchronised manner in 4–10 cycles per minute and involve all muscles of the body [6, 7]. Thanks to muscular activity, metabolic heat generation increases by 50–100%, and overall thermal condition of the body usually improves [8]. Shivering is considered organism's last line of defence against hypothermia.

Clinical signs

In its "natural" course, hypothermia, after an initial stimulation, leads to a gradual depression of almost all bodily systems [9]. Particular clinical stages of hypothermia are assigned approximate core temperature ranges, but clinical appearance and intensity of particular signs may individually vary – often depending on behavioural and cultural factors, circumstances, and accompanying disorders. Cases of individuals (e.g. climbers) who performed complicated activity in state of severe hypothermia are known. There are no laboratory tests helpful in diagnosis, differentiation, and staging of hypothermia. Function tests of most of organs show disorders proportional to severity and duration of hypothermia [3, 9]. Ability to interpret test results upon which clinical decisions are made may be crucial.

Hypothermia influences acid-base homeostasis in a specific and powerful manner. With drop of body temperature solubility of oxygen and carbon dioxide in plasma increases and activity of imidazole rings of histidine contained in haemoglobin becomes more pronounced. It is estimated that in closed system pH increases 0.015 units per each degree of drop of temperature in °C (Rosenthal correction factor). As a result, pH rises and partial pressure of carbon dioxide usually decreases already in an early phase of hypothermia. Further cooling usually entails metabolic acidosis resulting from peripheral hypoperfusion as well as cardiac and hepatic insufficiencies. Controversies concerning temperature correction in acid-base homeostasis testing exist. Diagnostic devices posses measurement (calculation) capability at current body temperature of the patient. Currently, the prevailing opinion states that in adults an uncorrected measurement should be performed, that is at 37°C (alfa-stat), whilst in children a corrected one is recommended (pH-stat) [10, 11]. Treatment of acid-base disorders based strictly on uncorrected values may lead to hyperventilation and cerebral hypoperfusion, whereas relying on corrected values may lead to hypercapnia, increase in cerebral perfusion, and brain *oedema* [12]. The choice of disorders interpretation method should depend on preferences and experience of a given centre. It should be noted that difference between arterial (uncorrected) partial pressure of CO_2 and end-tidal (EtCO_2) – at normothermia roughly 5 mmHg – increases already in moderate hypothermia up to approximately 15 mmHg. Establishing parameters of mechanical ventilation solely on EtCO_2 may thus be risk-laden. It should be emphasised that acid-base disorders rarely necessitate treatment – rewarming brings their spontaneous normalisation. It should also be stated that large volumes of 0.9% NaCl used in fluid resuscitation may aggravate acidosis. For this reason, and for reasons described above, intravenous fluids should be chosen in accordance with current laboratory test results [3].

Serum potassium level may undergo fast changes, especially during rewarming and fluctuations of acid-base balance. Hypokalaemia usually occurs in moderate hypothermia, and is caused by renal elimination of potassium and alkalosis. In more severe stages of hypothermia, hyperkalaemia results from acidosis and renal insufficiency [12]. Potassium level tends to be used as a prognostic factor in cases where hypothermia might have co-occurred with asphyxia [3, 13, 14]. If cardiac arrest took place in of water immersion or burial e.g. under snow and there are doubts concerning the sequence of events, plasma potassium level exceeding 12 mmol/L indicates occurrence of asphyxia before hypothermia. Potassium level lower than 10 mmol/L is a good prognostic, suggests occurrence of hypothermia before asphyxia, and – consequently – necessity to perform prolonged resuscitation until complete rewarming [3, 13, 14].

Caution is advocated during the rewarming process, as simultaneously with achieving normothermia and normalisation of acid-base disorders, potassium from intracellular space may undergo redistribution and hyperkalaemia may occur. This phenomenon is more often observed in acute post-exposure hypothermia when polyuria is less intense.

In chronic hypothermia (urban hypothermia) dehydration, haemoconcentration, and (often significantly) elevated hematocrit are likely. The fluid deficit is caused on one side by so called "cold diuresis," on the other by fluid distribution disorders, with fluid shift from intravascular space to extravascular one. Initial polyuria is caused by central overload resulting from peripheral vasoconstriction and reduced sensitivity of renal distant tubules to ADH [12]. Polyuria may be associated with hypomagesaemia and hypophosphataemia apart from hypokalaemia. In extreme forms of dehydration pre-renal kidney insufficiency may occur.

Hypothermia may also lead to glucose imbalances. Patients after acute exposure and who have shivered intensely may be expected to be hypoglycaemic. Thermogenesis by shivering is extremely "fuel-demanding"; full reserves of muscle and hepatic glycogen sustain shivers only for about 6 hours. After depletion of reserves, the shivers disappear with simultaneous emergence of tendency to hypoglycaemia aggravating to neuroglycopenia. On the other hand, patients who had undergone prolonged exposure may show tendency to hyperglycaemia. It is caused by decreased insulin secretion and peripheral insulin resistance resulting directly from hypothermia. It is worth noting that hyperglycaemia may aggravate polyuria and lead to water and electrolyte disturbances more severe than in hypothermia alone [12].

Interpretation of blood coagulation tests has been described in Chapter 14.

Treatment

Depending on both equipment availability as well as knowledge and creativity of the personnel there are several rewarming methods of various configurations used in practice [3].

In prehospital phase, prevention of further heat loss, avoidance of factors destabilising labile homeostasis and, if needed, provision of proper standard of resuscitation and transport to appropriate medical centre are essential. Attempts of aggressive rewarming are usually inefficient and may even be dangerous at this phase [3, 9, 13–15]. Patients in stage 4 of hypothermia (cardiac arrest) should be transported directly to facilities equipped with extracorporeal rewarming technology and possessing experience in such treatment. Use of devices for continuous mechanical chest compressions should be considered in transport of hypothermic patients in cardiac arrest [17, 18].

Choice of rewarming method in a hospital depends on local experience and availability of equipment. In most patients, even those in severe hypothermia, rewarming with passive and active, minimally invasive methods enables stable and safe rate of rewarming [3, 19, 20]. In patients in stage 3 who are hypotensive and/or suffering from ventricular arrhythmias as well as patients in stage 4 extracorporeal rewarming (ECR) with ECMO or CPB is recommended. Additional advantage of ECR is capability to sustain organ perfusion during rewarming even in patients in cardiac arrest [3, 21, 22].

Traditional recommendations dating from 1960's and 1970's advocate that rate of rewarming in hypothermia, especially in accompanying hypotension, should not exceed 0.5°C per hour [23]. Such "cautious" recommendations were aiming to prevent pulmonary and cerebral oedema as well as reduce the risk of circulatory failure. Too slow a process of rewarming, however, may be a factor increasing a risk of death. It appears that availability of increasingly advanced and efficient methods of rewarming as well as amelioration of capabilities to monitor the patient and provide intensive care made 1–1.5°C per hour an optimal and safe rate of rewarming.

Early phase of treatment of patients in severe hypothermia (HT 3) is burdened with risks of grave complications. Irruptive manipulations and interventions may aggravate hypovolaemia, intensify acid-base balance disorders, arrhythmias, and cause cardiac arrest. The so called "rescue collapse" syndrome may complicate rewarming at any phase of treatment [24]. Another danger is so called "afterdrop," defined as (often sudden) drop of core temperature after initiation of external rewarming. Clinical importance of this phenomenon is disputed nowadays [3].

Prognosis

Mortality rate in hypothermia amounts to 20–90% and depends on stage and type of hypothermia, coexisting disorders, and, most likely, on method of rewarming [19–22, 25, 26]. In acute primary hypothermia, if no cardiac arrest occurred, prognosis is usually good. Death caused solely by hypothermia occurs most often during rewarming – within 24 hours from admittance to hospital. For the patients in secondary hypothermia who have survived that stage, the following 48 hours are critical, during which symptoms of multi-organ failure emerge (which result usually from aggravation of coexisting diseases). For this reason it is recommended that treatment is conducted in intensive care units, in conditions enabling complex haemodynamic monitoring, and, if needed, implementation of invasive methods of rewarming [19–22].

References

1. Guly H. History of accidental hypothermia. Resuscitation 2011; 82: 122–125.
2. Kosiński S., Darocha T., Gałązkowski R. et al. Accidental hypothermia in Poland – estimation of prevalence, diagnostic methods and treatment. Scand. J. Trauma Resusc. Emerg. Med. 2015; 23: 13, doi: 10.1186/s13049-014-0086-7.
3. Brown D.J., Brugger H., Boyd J. et al. Accidental hypothermia. N. Engl. J. Med. 2012; 367: 1930–1938.

4. Danzl D.F., Pozos S.R. *Accidental hypothermia*. N. Engl. J. Med. 1994; 331: 1756–1760.

5. Giesbrecht G.G., Wilkerson J.A. *Hypothermia, frostbite and other cold injuries: prevention, survival, rescue, and treatment*. The Mountaineers Books, Seattle, USA 2006.

6. Sessler D.I. *Thermoregulatory defence mechanisms*. Crit. Care Med. 2009; 37(suppl): 203–210.

7. Sessler D.I. *Perioperative heat balance*. Anesthesiology 2000; 92: 578–596.

8. Frank S.M. *Consequences of hypothermia*. Curr. Anesth. Crit. Care 2001; 12: 79–86.

9. Kempainen R.R., Brunette D.D. *The evaluation and management of accidental hypothermia*. Respir. Care 2004; 49: 192–205.

10. Ashwood E.R., Kost G., Kenny M. *Temperature correction of blood-gas and pH measurements*. Clin. Chem. 1983; 29: 1877–1885.

11. Aziz K.A.A., Meduoye A. *Is pH-stat or alpha-stat the best technique to follow in patients undergoing deep hypothermic circulatory arrest?* Interact. Cardiovasc. Thorac. Surg. 2010; 10: 271–282.

12. Poldermann K. *Mechanisms of action, physiological effect and complications of hypothermia*. Crit. Care Med. 2009; 37: 186–202.

13. Durrer B., Brugger H., Syme D. *The medical on-site treatment of hypothermia ICAR-MEDCOM recommendation*. High Alt. Med. Biol. 2003; 4: 99–10.

14. Soar J., Perkins G.D., Abbas G. et al. *European Resuscitation Council Guidelines for Resuscitation 2010 Section 8. Cardiac arrest in special circumstances: Electrolyte abnormalities, poisoning, drowning, accidental hypothermia, hyperthermia, asthma, anaphylaxis, cardiac surgery, trauma, pregnancy, electrocution*. Resuscitation 2010; 81: 1400–1433.

15. Mulcahy A., Watts M.R. *Accidental hypothermia: an evidence-based approach*. Emerg. Med. Pract. 2009; 11: 1–23.

16. Alfonzo A., Lomas A., Drummond I. et al. *Survival after 5-h resuscitation attempt for hypothermic cardiac arrest using CVVH for extracorporeal rewarming*. Nephrol. Dial. Transplant. 2009; 24: 1054–1056.

17. Holmström P., Boyd J., Sorsa M. et al. *A case of hypothermic cardiac arrest treated with an external chest compression device (LUCAS) during transport to re-warming*. Resuscitation 2005; 67: 139–141.

18. Kosiński S., Jasiński J., Krzeptowski-Sabała S. et al. *AutoPulse w ratownictwie górskim – opis zastosowania urządzenia podczas śmigłowcowej ewakuacji ofiary lawiny*. Anestezjol. Ratown. 2013; 7: 310–313.

19. Roeggla M., Holzer M., Roeggla G. et al. *Prognosis of accidental hypothermia in the urban setting*. J. Intens. Care Med. 2001; 16: 142–149.

20. Megarbane B., Axler O., Chary I. et al. *Hypothermia with indoor occurrence is associated with a worse outcome*. Intens. Care Med. 2000; 26: 1843–1849.

21. Farstad M., Andersen K.S., Koller M.E. et al. *Rewarming from accidental hypothermia by extracorporeal circulation: a retrospective study.* Eur. J. Cardiothorac. Surg. 2001; 20: 58–64.

22. Ruttmann E., Weissenbacher A., Ulmer H. et al. *Prolonged extracorporeal membrane oxygenation-assisted support provides improved survival in hypothermic patients with cardiocirculatory arrest.* J. Thorac. Cardiovasc. Surg. 2007; 134: 594–600.

23. Lloyd E.L. *Accidental hypothermia.* Resuscitation 1996; 32: 111–112.

24. Kosiński S., Janczy J., Kałuża D. *Przypadek głębokiej przypadkowej hipotermii w górach – opis postępowania ratowniczego i medycznego.* Med. Intens. Ratunk. 2007; 10(4): 239–242.

25. Hislop L.J., Wyatt J.P., McNueghton G.W. et al. *Urban hypothermia in the West of Scotland.* BMJ 1995; 311: 725–727.

26. Durakowic Z., Misigoj-Durakowic M., Corovic N. et al. *Urban hypothermia and hyperglycemia in the elderly.* Coll. Antropol. 2000; 24: 405–409.

2

Epidemiology and Estimating Preventable Deaths in Accidental Hypothermia

Agata Smoleń[1], Halina Piecewicz-Szczęsna[1], Małgorzata Bała[2,3]

[1] Chair and Department of Epidemiology and Clinical Research Methodology, Medical University of Lublin, Poland
[2] Department of Hygiene and Dietetics, Jagiellonian University, Cracow, Poland
[3] Systematic Reviews Unit-Polish Cochrane Branch, Jagiellonian University, Cracow, Poland

Introduction

Accidental hypothermia is one of major challenges faced by today's medicine. Medical professionals dealing with hypothermic patients experience practical difficulties in every phase of treatment of the disorder. Shortage of efficient means of measurement in prehospital phase results in difficulties in diagnosis. Dilemmas concerning qualification to particular rewarming methods follow. Reliable medical data upon which efficacy of medical actions can be estimated is scarce, whilst accepted protocols are based usually on clinical observations or opinions of experts. Many of these issues are caused directly or indirectly by shortage of reliable epidemiological indicators. Without knowing the actual size of the problem we are unable to assign adequate importance to hypothermia nor determine the priorities of planned actions.

Incidence, mortality and fatality rates

To assess epidemiological situation, negative population health measures are used, these include: incidence rate, mortality rate and fatality rate.

Incidence rate, or the risk of occurrence of a disease in a population, states the number of people who are affected by the disease (number of new incidences of the disease) in a given period of observation (e.g. a year) divided by population at risk (100,000 or 10,000 people in a population is often utilised) [1]. Incidence rate is an important measure of health situation of a population. Monitoring of incidence rate enables assessment of changes in different time periods and makes early response to needs possible. It is also a helpful indicator taken into consideration when planning means of treatment and prevention of disease occurrences.

Number of deaths and population on a given area allow to calculate death-related indicators. Mortality and fatality rates should not be mistaken. Mortality rate is a number of deaths caused by a given disease in a given time period (e.g. a year) divided by population at risk (per 100,000 or 10,000 people in a population) in the studied time period. On the other hand, fatality rate is a ratio of deaths caused by a given disease and sum of all suffering from it (treated and deceased) in an analysed period of observation [1]. Fatality rate is often used when measuring health condition of a given population and when taking actions aiming at its reduction. Maintaing appropriate registers of people suffering from certain disease and evaluation of number of the patients who are likely to die as a result of the disease allow not only for monitoring of likely deaths but also for planning of places and means of treatment. Determining the demand for highly specialised medical centres staffed with appropriately qualified personnel and possessing right equipment may be conducive to decrease in number of deaths.

According to the official statistical reports, occurrence/incidence/prevalence of hypothermia in Poland is relatively low and limited to autumn and winter seasons. In reality, the disorder probably occurs more often than is reported as there is a shortage of factual data concerning of hypothermia, particularly concerning secondary and post-traumatic hypothermia types.

Statistical data of General Police Headquarters of Poland are a valuable source of information. The data shows that from January to March 2015 hypothermia caused 32 deaths in Poland, in year 2014 it was 98 deceased (mortality rate was approximating 0.26 per 100,000 people in population), in year 2013 – 115 deceased (0.3 per 100,000). Study of period from October to March shows in 2012/2013 – 178 deaths, in 2013/2014 – 75 deaths, 2014/2015 – 74 deaths [2]. Summarising the data from the Police reports it can be stated that in years 2009–2013 (in October–March periods) hypothermia caused 853 deaths in Poland [3].

Another source of statistical information are data from Central Statistical Office of Poland. The analysis of death certificates issued in years 2009–2013 in the territory of Poland has shown that exposure to excessive natural cold was a primary cause of death of 2,198 persons, and average mortality rate per 100,000 citizens was 1.14. According to official data from Central Statistical Office, number of deaths caused by hypothermia in Poland is uneven (340 to 615 per year) and calculated fatality rate fluctuates from 0.88 to 1.60 per 100,000 citizens per year (Table 1) [4]. As a comparison, in United States hypothermia causes 1,500 deaths per year [5]. It is estimated however that the true number may be far greater [6].

Table 1. Deaths resulting from exposure to excessive natural cold in years 2009–2013 in Poland

Year	Number of deaths	Mortality rate per 100,000 citizens
2009	454	1.19
2010	615	1.60
2011	340	0.88
2012	427	1.11
2013	362	0.94
Total (2009–2013)	2,198	average value: 1.14

Source: *Deaths in Poland in years 2009–2013*. Central Statistical Office of Poland, Warszawa 2015 [4].

An important source of information are data originating from medical institutions in Poland, which are collected on the basis of direct involvement of medical staff and patients. According to a large questionnaire survey conducted by Kosiński et al. in 50 emergency wards in Poland (with over 5.3 million citizens of Poland assigned/under care) incidence rate of clinically important accidental hypothermia is estimated to be 5.05 cases per 100,000 citizens per year. Fatality rate in the in the studied group was 6.3%. The authors emphasise however that the value includes only hypothermic patients treated in emergency wards (patients transferred from emergency wards to other wards were not monitored). In the studied group the most prevalent cause of hypothermia was exposure to cold air (87.3% of the studied population, 67.9% of which were alcohol abusers), only 6% of the cases were related to cold water immersion [6].

It is worth noting that in many regions where risk of hypothermia is theoretically low, temperature measurement is practiced rarely and shortages of specialised equipment allow only for measurement of peripheral temperature. A significant problem may be represented by urban hypothermia, which concerns inhabitants of cities, in particular the elderly affected by chronic health disorders [3, 7].

Preventable deaths in hypothermia

In 1976 a team lead by David D. Rutstein has devised an interesting and innovatory concept of assessment of medical care standards. The term "preventable death" introduced then stands for premature death resulting from selected causes which can be prevented by use of appropriate diagnostics, methods of treatment, and/or appropriate means of prevention [8].

Among 2,198 deceased on account of hypothermia in years 2009–2013, 624 (28.4%) were pronounced dead in hospitals. Consequently, this group should be considered as preventable deaths (Table 2).

Present experience of Severe Hypothermia Treatment Centre (SHTC) in Krakow shows that severe hypothermia (at least III in Swiss Staging Scale) is a classic example of disorder in which mortality can be significantly reduced, provided that appropriate treatment is implemented early enough [3].

Analysis of literature has allowed to identify two major factors directly related to premature deaths: lack of correct diagnosis and lack of appropriate treatment. Other important factors are: delay in diagnosis and/or delay in commencement of treatment, bad coordination of actions on various levels of medical care and availability of specialised treatment [8–12].

Table 2. Deaths resulting from hypothermia in years 2009–2013 including the place of death

Year	Number of deaths	Place of death			
		in hospital	in other medi-cal institution	at home	in other place
2009	454	105	1	64	284
2010	615	164	4	85	362
2011	340	99	2	44	195
2012	427	121	2	68	236
2013	362	135	0	29	198
Total (2009–2013)	2,198	624	9	290	1,275

Source: *Deaths in Poland in years 2009–2013*. Central Statistical Office of Poland, Warszawa 2015 [4].

Rare causes of disorders, including accidental hypothermia, are the very instances where amelioration of all above mentioned elements may bring desired results. SHTC in Kraków does not concentrate only on methods of treatment, but also its availability (i.e. awareness of existence of the treatment), as early as possible identification of hypothermic patients, and establishing rules of early treatment and transportation of patient. The system, created from scratch, is constantly modified upon acquired experience. In each solution like this (e.g. chain of survival in cardiac arrest) each phase (link of the chain) must be succinctly defined and emerge as a consequence of the previous one. Yet first of all, in order to be efficient such system must be functional, that is adapted to reality of medical practice. We hope that solutions developed by SHTC in Kraków will eventually become implemented in other regions of Poland.

It is a generally accepted rule that hypothermic patients in III or IV (Swiss Staging System) stage of hypothermia with clinically present circulatory instability and body temperature < 28°C are treated with extracorporeal circulation [3, 5]. The benefits of this modern method of treatment seem obvious. Isolation of high risk groups as well as early implementation of the treatment with extracorporeal circulation may aid in reduction of number of deaths caused by hypothermia. Extracorporeal rewarming is an invasive, but thanks to a proper organisation, available treatment for the patients in the most severe stages of hypothermia.

Survey of research on use of extracorporeal blood rewarming

In 2014 a systematic review was published in which extracorporeal rewarming (ECR) in severe hypothermia (core temperature < 28°C) was assessed [13]. The analysis comprised one study with control group [14], 12 case series and 15 case studies. The results concerning survival and neurological condition of patients upon discharge from hospital (according to definition in the studies) were presented in Table 3.

Because the above-mentioned review involved research published up to 2012, and from that year many new studies have appeared, another, authors'/proprietary, analysis of Medline and Embase databases was conducted. 39 articles published in 2012 or later were identified. Five studies were presented as conference materials – two of which were later published as clinical studies [15–17]. In two references no information regarding hypothermia or separate results concerning hypothermic patients were provided. Moreover, in two studies body temperature of patients was above 28°C, in one study ECR was not implemented, in one hypothermia was caused by poisoning. Eventually the analysis included 9 case series and 10 case studies. The results concerning survival and neurological condition (according to definition in the studies) were presented in Tables 3 and 4. Data on patients in severe hypothermia (core temperature < 28°C) were isolated from studies discussing mainly cases of mild and moderate stages of hypothermia (> 28°C). Table 4 includes also the results of studies in which no temperature in hypothermic patients rewarmed with ECR was provided.

In 10 studies 13 cases of hypothermia treated with ECR were described – 9 concerned adults, 4 children or adolescents. The results were presented in Table 5.

It is difficult to draw conclusions about efficacy of ECR in severe hypothermia upon the retrieved publications. All studies except one were case series or case studies. Hence all of them were characterised by high risk of systematic error. Rapidly growing bulk of data implies usefulness of

Table 3. Results of studies included in systematic survey

Type od study	Number of patients with ECR implemented (number of of patients assessed for neurological condition, if varied)	Sub-group[a,b]	Total survival	Positive neurological condition/good neurological outcome
study with control group – adults [14]	68	–	84.2% in ECR group, 46.6% in control group	no data
case series – children and adults (12 sudies) [13]	141 (127)	asphyxia[a] (11 studies)	33 (23.4%)	12 (9.4%)
	90 (52)	exposure to cold[b] (7 sudies)	61 (67.7%)	32 (61.5%)
including case series and case studies only concerning children (8 studies) [13]	56	asphyxia[a]	15 (26.8%)	7 (12.5%)
	1	cold[b]	1	1
case studies concerning adults (15 studies) [13]	3	asphyxia[a]	3	3
	14	cold[b]	14	14

[a] cardiac arrest caused by asphyxia with accompanying hypothermia (drowning, avalanche victims)
[b] cardiac arrest caused by exposure to cold

Source: Own compilation upon Dunne B. et al. *Extracorporeal-assisted rewarming in the management of accidental deep hypothermic cardiac arrest. A systematic review of the literature. Heart Lung Circ.* 2014; 23(11): 1029–1035 [13].

ERC treatment of patients in severe stages of hypothermia, particularly in cardiac arrest. The analyses confirm the relatively rare implementation of ECR and existence of a small group of specialists dealing with the issue.

So as to obtain a broad set of information regarding accidental hypothermia, professor Beat Walpoth of University Hospital of Geneva has initiated International Hypothermia Registry (www.hypothermia-registry.org) in which Kraków's SHTC also participates. We hope that thanks to this fact fuller and more detailed information about hypothermia and means of treatment will soon be available.

Table 4. Application of ECR in hypothermia – case series studies published in years 2012–2015

Study (authors' names)	Number of patients with ECR implemented – total and in sub-groups (core body temperature)	Cause of hypothermia	Total survival	Positive neurological condition
Agersnap 2012 [18]	7 adolescents (15.5–24°C)	exposure to cold water	7/7	no data
Boue 2014a [19]	21[a] (no data)	avalanche	3/21	3/21
Darocha 2015a [20]	9 (23.6 ± 3.3°C one patient 29°C)	exposure to cold	9/9	9/9
Debaty 2015 [21]	23 (no data)[b]	avalanche, drowning, exposure to cold	9/23	no data
Jarosz 2015 [21]	4 (22.2–25.7°C)[c]	exposure to cold	4/4	4/4
Mair 2014 [23]	28 (no data)	avalanche	2	2
Mochizuki 2014 [15–17]	7 (no data)	no data	5/7	5/7
Moroder 2015 [24]	4d (22–28°C)	avalanche	0/4	–
Sawamoto 2014 [25]	26 (median 24.4°C)	near-drowning (submersion), avalanche, cold exposure	26/26	10/26

[a] not provided for patients undergoing ECR, for the entire group 28.0°C (26.0–30.7)
[b] not provided for patients undergoing ECR, for the entire group 26.0°C (24.0–27.2)
[c] the study includes one more hypothermia case (32°C), caused by exposure to cold water, treated with ECR, resulting in death
[d] 4 (out of 23 described) had ECR implemented

Source: Authors' own compilation.

Table 5. Application of ECR in hypothermia – case studies published in years 2012–2015

Case studies	Number of patients with ECR implemented (core body temperature)	Cause of hypothermia	Total survival	Positive neurological condition
		adults		
Boue 2014b [26]	2 (21.1°C)	avalanche	2	2
Boue 2014c [27]	1 (16.9°C)	exposure to cold	1	1
Darocha 2015b [28]	1 (25°C)	exposure to cold	1	1
Hungerer 2013 [29]	1 (23°C)	exposure to cold	1	0
Mark 2012 [30]	1 (27.5°C)	exposure to cold water	1	1
Meyer 2014 [31]	1 (20.8°C)	exposure to cold water	1	1
Morley 2013 [33]	1 (< 25°C)	exposure to cold	1	1
Nordberg 2014 [33]	1 (22°C)	exposure to cold	1	1
		adolescents and children		
Hungerer 2013 [29]	one adolescent	exposure to cold	0	0
Jane 2013 [34]	two children (< 30°C)	exposure to cold water	1	0
Romlin 2015 [35]	one child (13.8°C)	exposure to cold water	1	1

Source: Authors' own compilation.

References

1. *Leksykon epidemiologiczny*, ed. J. Bzdęga, W. Magdzik, D. Naruszewicz-Lesiuk, A. Zieliński. Wyd. a-Medica Press, Bielsko-Biała 2008.

2. *Statystyka-zgonów-z-powodu-wychłodzenia* (http://statystyka.policja.pl/st/wolny tekst/60372; accessed: 7.10.2015).

3. Darocha T., Kosiński S., Jarosz A. et al. *Zasady postępowania w wychłodzeniu – małopolski program pozaustrojowego leczenia hipotermii.* Kardiol. Pol. 2015; 73(9): 789–794.

4. *Zgony w latach 2009–2013 na terenie Polski.* Centralne Informatorium GUS, Warszawa 2015.

5. Brown D.J., Brugger H., Boyd J. *Accidental hypothermia.* N. Engl. J. Med. 2012; 367: 1930–1938.

6. Kosiński S., Darocha T., Gałązkowski R. et al. *Accidental hypothermia in Poland – estimation of prevalence, diagnostic methods and treatment.* Scand. J. Trauma Resusc. Emerg. Med. 2015; 23: 13.

7. Kosiński S., Górka A. *Specyfika i czynniki ryzyka miejskiej postaci hipotermii.* Anestezjol. Ratown. 2010; 4: 239–249.

8. Rutstein D.D., Berenberg W., Chalmers T.C. et al. *Measuring the Quality of Medical Care. A Clinical Method.* N. Engl. J. Med. 1976; 294(11): 582–588.

9. Westerling R., Gullberg A., Rosen M. *Socioeconomic differences in 'avoidable' mortality in Sweden, 1986–1990.* Int. J. Epidemiol. 1996; 25: 560–567.

10. WHO. *The World Health Report 2000. Health Systems: Improving performance.* World Health Organization, Genewa 2000.

11. Nolte E., McKee M. *Variations in amenable mortality – trends in 16 high-income nations.* Health Policy 2011; 103(1): 47–52.

12. Wróblewska W. *Zgony możliwe do uniknięcia – opis koncepcji oraz wyniki analizy dla Polski.* Studia Demogr. 2012; 1(161): 129–151.

13. Dunne B., Christou E., Duff O. et al. *Extracorporeal-assisted rewarming in the management of accidental deep hypothermic cardiac arrest. A systematic review of the literature.* Heart Lung Circ. 2014; 23(11): 1029–1035.

14. Morita S., Inokuchi S., Yamagiwa T. et al. *Efficacy of portable and percutaneous cardiopulmonary bypass rewarming versus that of conventional internal rewarming for patients with accidental deep hypothermia.* Crit. Care Med. 2011; 39(5): 1064–1068.

15. Mochizuki K., Imamura H. *Extracorporeal cardiopulmonary resuscitation with cardiac arrest bypass system for refractory out-of-hospital cardiac arrest is associated with favorable survival.* Circulation 2014; 130: A12316.

16. Mochizuki K., Imamura H., Iwashita T. et al. *Neurological outcomes after extracorporeal cardiopulmonary resuscitation in patients with out-of-hospital cardiac arrest: a retrospective observational study in a rural tertiary care center.* J. Intens. Care 2014; 2(1): 33.

17. Mochizuki K. et al. *Extracorporeal cardiopulmonary resuscitation for refractory out-of-hospital cardiac arrest is associated with favorable survival: Possible indications.* Circulation 2012; 126(21).

18. Agersnap L. et al. *6 months outcome after severe accidental hypothermia and cardiac arrest in 7 teenagers.* Neurorehabil. Neural Repair 2012; 26(4): 412.

19. Boué Y., Paven P.J., Brun J., Thomas S. et al. *Survival after avalanche-induced cardiac arrest.* Resuscitation 2014; 85(9): 1192–1196, doi: 10.1016/j.resuscitation. 2014.06.015. Epub 2014 Jun 24, 2014.

20. Darocha T., Sobczyk D., Kosinski S. et al. *New diastolic cardiomyopathy in patients with severe accidental hypothermia after ECMO rewarming: A case-series observational study.* Cardiovasc. Ultrasound. 2015; 13(1).

21. Debaty G., Moustapha I., Bouzat P. et al. *Outcome after severe accidental hypothermia in the French Alps: A 10-year review.* Resuscitation 2015; 93: 118–123.

22. Jarosz A., Darocha T., Kosiński S. et al. *Extracorporeal membrane oxygenation in severe accidental hypothermia.* Intens. Care Med. 2014; 41(1): 169–170.

23. Mair P., Brugger H., Mair B. et al. *Is extracorporeal rewarming indicated in avalanche victims with unwitnessed hypothermic cardiorespiratory arrest?* High Alt. Med. Biol. 2014; 15(4): 500–503.

24. Moroder L., Mair B., Brugger H. et al. *Outcome of avalanche victims with out-of-hospital cardiac arrest.* Resuscitation 2015; 89(C): 114–118.

25. Sawamoto K., Bird S.B., Katayama Y. et al. *Outcome from severe accidental hypothermia with cardiac arrest resuscitated with extracorporeal cardiopulmonary resuscitation.* Am. J. Emerg. Med. 2014; 32(4): 320–324.

26. Boué Y., Paven J.F., Torres J.P., Blancher M., Bouzat P. *Full Neurologic Recovery after Prolonged Avalanche Burial and Cardiac Arrest.* High Alt. Med. Biol. 2014; 15(4): 522–523, doi: 10.1089/ham.2014.1082, 2014.

27. Boue Y., Lavolaine J., Bouzat P. et al. *Neurologic recovery from profound accidental hypothermia after 5 hours of cardiopulmonary resuscitation.* Crit. Care Med. 2014; 42(2): e167–e170.

28. Darocha T., Kosiński S., Jarosz A. et al. *Extracorporeal Rewarming From Accidental Hypothermia of Patient With Suspected Trauma.* Medicine (Baltimore) 2015; 94(27): e1086.

29. Hungerer S. et al. *Accidental, profound hypothermia in mountain rescue emergencies.* Notfall Rettungsmed. 2013; 16(2): 114–120.

30. Mark E.LJ.O., Kjerstad A., Naesheim T. et al. *Hypothermic cardiac arrest far away from the center providing rewarming with extracorporeal circulation.* Int. J. Emerg. Med. 2012; 5: 7, doi: 10.1186/1865-1380-5-7, 2012.

31. Meyer M., Pelurson N., Khabiri E. et al. *Sequela-free long-term survival of a 65-year-old woman after 8 hours and 40 minutes of cardiac arrest from deep accidental hypothermia.* J. Thorac. Cardiovasc. Surg. 2014; 147(1): e1–e2.

32. Morley D., Yamane K., O'Malley R. et al. *Rewarming for accidental hypothermia in an urban medical center using extracorporeal membrane oxygenation.* Am. J. Case Rep. 2013; 14: 6–9.
33. Nordberg P., Ivert T., Dalén M. et al. *Surviving two hours of ventricular fibrillation in accidental hypothermia.* Prehosp. Emerg. Care 2014; 18(3): 446–449.
34. Jane G. et al. *Extracorporeal cardiopulmonary resuscitation (ECPR) for paediatric out of hospital arrest.* Int. J. Art. Organs 2013; 36(4): 285.
35. Romlin B.S., Winberg H., Janson M. et al. *Excellent Outcome With Extracorporeal Membrane Oxygenation After Accidental Profound Hypothermia (13.8 degrees C) and Drowning.* Crit. Care Med. 2015; 43(11): e521–e525.

3

Facts and Myths about Hypothermia and its Treatment

Sylweriusz Kosiński[1,2,3], Tomasz Darocha[3,4]

[1] Department of Anesthesiology and Intensive Care, Pulmonary Hospital, Zakopane, Poland
[2] Tatra Mountain Rescue Service, Zakopane, Poland
[3] "Heat for Life" Foundation, Cracow, Poland
[4] Severe Hypothermia Treatment Centre, Department of Anaesthesiology and Intensive Care, John Paul II Hospital, Cracow, Poland

Human organism is able to adapt to extreme external conditions. Among other reasons, this characteristic has enabled humans to flourish on Earth. We are generally able to fight cold, but in some conditions this defence proves inefficient. And even though our knowledge of hypothermia is constantly becoming more comprehensive, many doubts, myths and understatements pertaining to this phenomenon persist. We would like to make an attempt here to clarify some of them.

Hypothermia and "freezing with cold" are not the same thing

Common "freezing with cold" means exposure to cold, but it does not necessarily mean lowering of core body temperature. We speak of hypothermia when temperature of internal organs of the body drops below 35°C (Table 1). If a cause of drop in temperature is a simple disproportion between heat generation and loss, we speak about "accidental hypothermia." If hypothermia is caused by body trauma, we speak about "post-traumatic hypothermia." It is worth noting that post-traumatic hypothermia varies in many ways from accidental hypothermia, and different temperature thresholds are assigned to both types of the disorder (Table 1) [1, 2].

Table 1. Hypothermia classification

Classification	Accidental hypothermia	Post-traumatic hypothermia
mild	35–32°C	36–34°C
moderate	32–28°C	34–32°C
severe	< 28°C	< 32°C

Source: Own compiled upon American College of Surgeons Committee in Trauma. *Advanced Trauma Life Support for Doctors, Student Course Manual,* Eight Edition. American College of Surgeons 2008 [1].

Cold "creeps in" however it can

From a physical point of view, warmth may equally stand for both quantity as well as a form of internal energy transmission in a system [3]. If we say that an object is warm, it means it has a higher internal energy than the environment. So is the other way round: an object described as cold has lower internal energy. The process of heat transferral occurs between systems (bodies) of different temperatures – from the warmer system (of higher energy) to colder one (of lower energy). Hence, it is not the cold that "creeps in" but the warmth that "escapes."

Human beings lose most of their heat by radiating it outside

Human body dissipates heat by four processes: radiation, convection, conduction, and evaporation. In a closed room, with minimal air movement, and in standard room temperature (21°C), an undressed human indeed loses most of his/her heat (about 55%) as infrared radiation [4, 5]. But with increase of air movement convection becomes a prevalent heat loss process [4]. If we immerse the body in water or place it on cold surface – heat will be mostly lost by conduction [5–9]. On the other hand, in warm climate (where temperature of environment is approximately equal to body temperature), the primary heat loss process is sweat evaporation. From a practical point of view it is worth remembering that radiation is both a process of heat dissipation as well as its accumulation. During the day organism can absorb sun radiation which – if sufficiently intense – cancels out the heat loss and protects from hypothermia. No cover however can fully stop radiation. Reflective blankets such as aluminium foil reduce radiation loss only to a small degree [10–12].

Clothing stops the heat loss

Even if a person is dressed "head to toe," the heat is still lost. First of all, about 10% of total heat loss occurs with exhaled air [13]. Secondly, the kind and thickness of garment is important. It is hard to make a perfect barrier that would stop the heat loss processes in all conditions. Multi-layered, full clothing of entire body may start "leaking" when the body is supine. Part of clothing which is between the body and the ground (about 25% of body surface) becomes compressed, and thermic insulation becomes radically reduced. In such situation, a significant portion of heat starts to "escape" to the ground. Even the perfect clothing or cover ceases to serve its function when it becomes wet. Water collected in the structure of the fabric (e.g. sweat) and in direct contact with the body loses its warmth by means of convection, and also by evaporation. The heat loss via wet piece of clothing is a few times greater than by the same, but dry one [6–8, 14].

Half of total body heat is lost via head

A human dressed in arctic, almost perfectly insulating clothing who has his hat taken off in an extremely cold environment may indeed lose half of the total heat emitted to the environment (including heat loss via airways) via head [15]. But in normal conditions the loss of heat should not exceed the amount corresponding to body surface (that is about 10–15%) [16, 17].

It should be noted however that head can be a source of significant heat loss as a result of physiological processes. Cutaneous blood vessels of the head do not become constricted (or constrict only to a limited degree) in cold environment, as the proper blood supply to the brain is a vital priority of the organism [18]. If blood vessels of other body parts become constricted, the heat loss may be somewhat greater than is implied by body surface.

The best protection from cold is metallised rescue blanket

Metallised thermal blankets are light, strong and durable, but belief in their exceptional qualities is unjustified. The reflective layer of the blanket is supposed to "return the heat" which is being radiated by the body. It turned out, however, that thermic insulation qualities of such blankets are similar to any other material of comparable thickness [10, 12, 19]. Thermal blankets are excellent as an external layer of multiple layer insulation (thanks to their wind- and waterproofness), but worn directly on body they provide mediocre thermal barrier [12].

Hypothermia happens only in wintertime

Hypothermia may occur everywhere in the world, in any season of the year [20]. Naturally, the colder the environment, the greater the risk of hypothermia. It should be kept in mind that hypothermia occurs when energetic balance within organism is negative (that is when we lose more heat than we produce). So, when heat production, for any reason, is impaired, even a normal heat loss leads to gradual hypothermia. It is assumed that deficit of 85 kcal (which equals to energy produced in an hour) may cause a drop of body temperature by up to 1°C [21]. That is how so-called "urban hypothermia" develops. Shortage of even a few kcal per 24 hours accumulates, and emerging clinical signs are masked by adaptation mechanisms [20].

Hypothermia is nothing to worry about as it is used also for therapeutic reasons

Both types of unintended hypothermia are fatal disorders, untreated may lead to death [22, 23]. Drop of core body temperature below 28°C may cause grave heart arrhythmias or severe bradycardia leading eventually to cardiac arrest. Hypothermia occurring after body injuries aggravates circulatory disorders, disturbs coagulation and metabolism, making the prognosis much worse [23, 24]. Therapeutic hypothermia, practiced after successful resuscitation or after neurosurgeries is induced in hospital, under strict control, and should not be mistaken with unintended hypothermia.

Any thermometer is good when measuring body temperature

In hypothermia, the core (or central) body temperature measurement is considered the optimal method, as it reflects the temperature of internal body organs. As a consequence of anastomoses contraction the difference between "core" and "shell" (that is between the central and peripheral areas of the body) increases, and the result of measurement in the armpit may differ several or even a dozen degrees from the temperature of the heart or the brain. For this reason, hypothermia is staged according to core temperature, which is best measured in the oesophagus, urinary bladder, rectum or tympanic membrane [25, 26].

Cold improves blood clotting

Hypothermia leads to coagulation disorders, that is why it poses a great danger for patients with body injuries. Although mild stage of hypothermia may be associated with increase of coagulation, drop of temperature below 34°C translates into quick deterioration of almost all elements of clotting cascade. These disorders are not treatable with pharmaceuticals, but can be reversed after rewarming of the patient [27].

Wet clothes should be taken of as soon as possible

Yes, but only in safe, warm and dry place. Even wet clothing provides some thermic insulation. For instance, fabric made from natural wool taken out of water insulates only 20% worse than dry one. One must also keep in mind that in harsh weather (e.g. strong wind, subzero cold) even a brief exposure of body deprived of cover causes rapid and massive loss of heat. If an impermeable, wind- and waterproof layer is applied (e.g. plastic wrap or metallised blanket) onto wet clothing the resulting heat loss is comparable to situation when clothing is removed and dry cover is applied [28, 29]. Removing the wet clothes of the patient should rather be delayed until the person is in, for instance, a heated interior of an ambulance. Until then it is recommended to put another thick, impermeable layer of fabric and insulate the patient from the ground. One should also note that even when wet clothing is cut before removal, and prior to dressing the patient in dry covers, it is difficult to avoid movements of the body and manual operations, which in severe hypothermia may induce grave arrhythmias.

Hypothermic patient must be rewarmed as soon as possible

Indications for fast rewarming are limited to severe hypothermia with circulatory instability and risk of cardiac arrest (or after cardiac arrest). In such situations, it is recommended to implement extracorporeal rewarming in order to increase core temperature to a level not endangered by severe arrhythmias [25, 26]. It must be emphasised that this method of rewarming demands most meticulous monitoring and application of specialised instruments. In practice, extracorporeal rewarming is conducted only in cardiac surgery centres. If the patient is in mild or moderate hypothermia, usually non-invasive rewarming is used – external heat, warm intravenous infusions, warm air ventilation. In such situations, slow and stable rate or achieving normothermia is preferred (1–2°C per hour), which reduces the risk of complications (such as secondary drop of core temperature – so called "afterdrop" and shock – "rewarming shock") [25, 30]. In prehospital period the safest choice is protection of the patient from further heat loss by means of impermeable, multi-layered cover and resorting to active rewarming only in extreme necessity.

Medical procedure in hypothermia appears to be simple, but even experienced members of medical staff may be surprised by phenomena we have not yet fully understood.

We hope we managed to clarify at least some misunderstandings and doubts.

References

1. American College of Surgeons Committee in Trauma. *Advanced Trauma Life Support for Doctors, Sudent Course Manual*, Eight Edition. American College of Surgeons 2008.
2. Soar J., Perkins G.D., Abbas G. et al. *European Resuscitation Council Guidelines for Resuscitation 2010 Section 8. Cardiac arrest in special circumstances: Electrolyte abnormalities, poisoning, drowning, accidental hypothermia, hyperthermia, asthma, anaphylaxis, cardiac surgery, trauma, pregnancy, electrocution*. Resuscitation 2010; 81: 1400–1433.
3. Halliday D., Resnick R., Walker J. *Podstawy fizyki*, vol. 2. Wydawnictwo Naukowe PWN, Warszawa 2006.
4. Nilsson A.L. *Blood flow, temperature, and heat loss of skin exposed to local radiative and convective cooling*. J. Invest. Dermatol. 1987; 88: 586–593.
5. Arens E., Zhang H. *The skin's role in human termoregulation and comfort. Thermal and moisture transport in fibrous materials*. Woodhead Publishing 2006.
6. Richards M.G.M., Meinander H., Broede P. et al. *Dry and wet heat transfer through clothing dependent on the clothing properties under cold conditions*. Int. J. Occup. Saf. Ergon. 2008; 14: 69–76.
7. Lotens W.A., Vandelinde F.J.G., Havenith G. *Effects of condensation in clothing on heat transfer*. Ergonomics 1995; 38: 1114–1131.
8. Farnworth B., Dolhan P.A. *Heat loss through wet clothing insulation*. Defence Research Establishment, Ottawa 1983.
9. Brauer A., Pacholik L., Perl T. et al. *Conductive heat exchange with a gel-coated circulating water mattress*. Anesth. Analg. 2004; 99: 1742–1746.
10. Light I.M., Norman J.N. *The thermal properties of a survival bag incorporating metallised plastic sheeting*. Aviat. Space Environ. Med. 1980; 51: 367–370.
11. Giesbrecht G.G., Wilkerson J.A. *Hypothermia, frostbite and other cold injuries: prevention, survival, rescue, and treatment*. The Mountaineers Books, Seattle, USA 2006.

12. Ennemoser O., Ambach W., Flora G. *Physical assessment of heat insulation rescue foils.* Int. J. Sports Med. 1988; 9: 179–182.

13. Burch G.E. *Study of water and heat loss from the respiratory tract of man; methods: a gravimetric method for the measurement of the rate of water loss; a quantitative method for the measurement of the rate of heat loss.* Arch. Intern. Med. 1945; 76: 308–314.

14. Bakkevig M.K., Nielsen R. *Impact of wet underwear on thermoregulatory responses and thermal comfort in the cold.* Ergonomics 1994; 37: 1375–1389.

15. *US Army Survival Manual: FM 21-76.* US Department of the Army, 1970: 148.

16. Pretorius T., Bristow G.K., Steinman A.M. et al. *Effects of whole head submersion in cold water on nonshivering humans.* J. Appl. Physiol. 2006; 101: 669–675.

17. Rasch W., Samson P., Cote J. et al. *Heat loss from the human head during exercise.* J. Appl. Physiol. 1985; 71: 590–595.

18. Froese G., Burton A.C. *Heat losses from the human head.* J. Appl. Physiol. 1957; 10: 235–241.

19. Henriksson O., Lundgren P., Kuklane K. et al. *Protection against cold in prehospital care: evaporative heat loss reduction by wet clothing removal or the addition of a vapor barrier – a thermal manikin study.* Prehosp. Disaster Med. 2012; 27: 53–58.

20. Kosinski S., Górka A. *Specyfika i czynniki ryzyka miejskiej postaci hipotermii.* Anestezjol. Ratown. 2010; 4: 468–481.

21. Sessler D.I. *Perioperative heat balance.* Anaesthesiology 2000; 92: 578–596.

22. Kempainen R.R., Brunette D.D. *The evaluation and management of accidental hypothermia.* Respir. Care 2004; 49: 192–205.

23. Trentzsch H., Huber-Wagner S., Hildebrand F. et al. *Hypothermia for prediction of death in severely injured blunt trauma patients.* Shock 2012; 37: 131–139.

24. Arthurs Z., Cuadrado D., Beekley A. et al. *The impact of hypothermia on trauma care at the 31st combat support hospital.* Am. J. Surg. 2006; 191: 610–614.

25. Brown D.J., Brugger H., Boyd J. et al. *Accidental hypothermia.* N. Engl. J. Med. 2012; 367: 1930–1938.

26. Soar J., Perkins G.D., Abbas G. et al. *European Resuscitation Council Guidelines for Resuscitation 2010 Section 8. Cardiac arrest in special circumstances: Electrolyte abnormalities, poisoning, drowning, accidental hypothermia, hyperthermia, asthma, anaphylaxis, cardiac surgery, trauma, pregnancy, electrocution.* Resuscitation 2010; 81: 1400–1433.

27. Rohrer M.J., Natale A.M. *Effect of hypothermia on the coagulation cascade.* Crit. Care Med. 1992; 20: 1402–1405.

28. Thomassen Ø., Færevik H., Østerås Ø. et al. *Comparison of three different prehospital wrapping methods for preventing hypothermia – a crossover study in humans.* Scand. J. Trauma Resusc. Emerg. Med. 2011; 19: 41, doi: 10.1186/1757-7241-19-41.

29. Henriksson O., Lundgren J.P., Kuklane K. et al. *Protection against cold in prehospital care-thermal insulation properties of blankets and rescue bags in different wind conditions.* Prehosp. Disaster Med. 2009; 24: 408–415.
30. Lloyd E.L. *Accidental hypothermia.* Resuscitation 1996; 32: 111–124.

4

Measurement of Patient's Body Temperature

Jacek Majkowski[1], Tomasz Sanak[1,2,3]

[1] "Heat for Life" Foundation, Cracow, Poland
[2] Department of Disaster Medicine and Emergency Care, Medical Jagiellonian University Collegium Medicum, Cracow, Poland
[3] Department of Battlefield Medicine, Military Institute of Medicine, Warsaw, Poland

A bit of history

The first medical thermometer, based on Gallileo's concept, was crafted by Sanctorius of Padua. The relevant information was published in 1612. Yet the person who popularised the use of temperature measurement of patients was a German physician, Carl Wunderlich. After having performed more than a million of measurements on 25,000 patients, he calculated the average temperature of a healthy person to be 37°C, and defined "fever" as body temperature exceeding 38°C.

Temperature scales

In Poland, as in many countries, Celsius scale is used in medical measurements. The other legally approved temperature scale in Poland is Kelvin. As Kelvin scale is base unit of SI system, the term "degree" does not apply to it. So, in order to express relationship between the two scales we can say: "Temperature 0 degrees Celsius is 273.15 Kelvin." The difference stems from the fact that in Celsius scale 0 was set as a point of freezing of water, whilst in Kelvin scale 0 is absolute zero – theoretically lowest possible temperature.

There are only five countries in the world where Fahrenheit scale is used instead of Celsius: The Bahamas, Belize, Cayman Islands, Palau and… United States of America. It is rumoured that German scientist Fahrenheit accepted as 0 in his scale the lowest temperature of winter season 1708/1709 in his hometown Gdańsk ($-17.8°C$). Similar scale to Fahrenheit, with 0 at absolute zero, is Rankine scale. Rømer, Delisle, Newton and Réaumur scales are nowadays almost extinct. Yet, in 1841 there were at least 18 temperature scales!

Temperature measurements

Temperature cannot be measured directly like length or weight. A sensor which changes its physical properties must be used, for instance:

- change of volume of liquid (classic glass thermometers, e.g. containing mercury);
- change in resistance (thermistor and resistance temperature detector – RTD);
- generation of electric voltage in place of contact of two metals (thermocouple);
- change of colour (liquid crystal thermometer);
- deformation of bimetals (thermostat);
- emission of heat radiation (pyrometer, infrared sensor – IR);
- change of parameters of semiconductor contactors (integrated circuit – IC).

After nearly three centuries since development of the first Fahrenheit mercury thermometer, Council of Europe in directive 76/769/EWG has banned production and sale of such type of thermometers from 9 April 2009 on. Let us therefore concentrate on electronic devices, functioning upon principle shown on Figure 1.

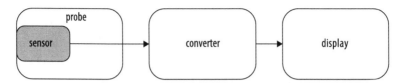

Figure 1. Schematic representation of electronic thermometer

Source: Study by Jacek Majkowski.

Important parameters of temperature sensors

Accuracy – degree of conformity of measured value to reality. If a thermometer has an accuracy of ± 0.1°C and presents value of 36.6°C it means the actual temperature may be equal to value between 36.5°C to 36.7°C. Accuracy is a characteristic of both sensor as well as of thermometer, for instance sensor can have accuracy of ± 0.05°C, but entire thermometer only ± 0.1°C. It is worth to mention another characteristic of a thermometer, yet not the sensor, which is resolution. In case of electronic devices it is the smallest number that can be read from the display, e.g. 0.01°C. It should be remembered however that that accuracy should not be confused with resolution. A thermometer with a cheap sensor of adequacy of 0.5°C can be equipped with a display of resolution of 0.01°C. The value of 36.86°C on display may in reality be both 36.36°C as well as 37.36°C.

Sensitivity – stands for the smallest change of temperature that can be recorded by a thermometer. In other words: how great a change of measured value (e.g. height of mercury column, resistance) is caused by change of temperature by 1°C.

Temperature range – stands for range of values for which a sensor guarantees accuracy. From a point of view of measuring human body temperature, and considering hypo- and hyperthermia, range of 10–50°C is desired. It should be noted that most medical thermometers have very narrow range, typically 35–42°C, insufficient for diagnosis of hypothermia.

Thermal response time – i.e. time necessary for measurement of a new value after sudden change of sensor's temperature, or, in other words,

Table 1. Comparison of popular temperature sensors

	Glass thermometer (mercury, alcohol, galinstan)	Thermistor	Metal resistance thermometer (platinum, nickel)	Thermocouple	Infrared sensors, pyrometers	Integrated circuit – IC
temperature range	from −200°C to +356°C (medical ones typically 35–42°C)	from −100°C to +500°C (typically from −80°C to +150°C)	from −260°C to +960°C	from −270°C to +2316°C	from −100°C to +500°C	from −55°C to +150°C
accuracy	++ (0,1°C)	++/+++	+++	++	+	0.1°C
reaction time (approximate time until stable reading)	+ (300 s)	+++ (5 s)	+	++	+++	+++ (5 s)
sensitivity	++	+++	++	+	++	++
cost	$	$	$$$	$$	$$	$
ruggedness	+	++	+	+++	+	++
advantages	popularity	highest sensitivity	highest accuracy, averaging of temperatures	highest temperatures	non-contact measurement	miniaturization (e.g. thermometers can be swallowed as a pill)

Source: Study by Jacek Majkowski.

how long one must wait for a result after the beginning of measurement of patient's body temperature. Time of response is also influenced by the material of the probe encapsulating the sensor.

Repeatability – i.e. what are the differences between consecutive measurements with different thermometers of the same type. High-end sensors provide reproducibility of ± 0.05°C in the entire range.

Ruggedness – means low vulnerability to mechanical damage, such as: shocks, crushes, water etc.

After analysis of data presented in Table 1 an attentive reader will probably conclude that the best sensor for measurement of patient's body temperature is thermistor – indeed it is the most popular sensor on medical market.

Review of thermistor medical probes

Market offers a broad range of certified probes for measurement of human body temperature (Figure 2), including:

- universal PVC tube probes, about 75 cm long, designed for measurements in oesophagus, rectum or nasopharynx;
- probes for tympanic membrane measurement with a tip of soft material adapting to shape of ear canal and blocking the air movement from outside (which could disturb the measurement), available also in children sizes;
- skin adhesive pads, also in neonatal sizes;
- probes for measurement in oesophagus with integrated stethoscope transmitting sounds of heart and lungs;
- probes integrated into Foley catheter for measurement in urinary bladder and proximal part of urethra;
- integrated into superfine needle for measurement of myocardium temperature during open-heart surgery.

Most of the probes are single use products delivered in sterile package.

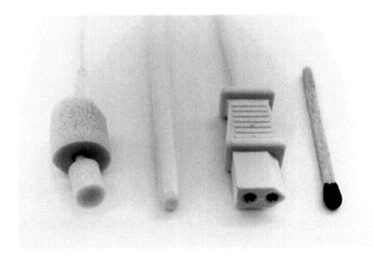

Figure 2. From left to right: tip of ear canal probe, tip of universal probe (rectal or oesophagal), plug of the probe to be attached to measuring apparatus, match – for size comparison

Source: Image by Jacek Majkowski.

Measurement duration

Time after which thermistor reaches the temperature of the measured body is given in time constant in seconds. It depends mainly on thermistor or probe size (the greater the size the longer the time thermic equilibrium with examined object is reached), material of the probe, and the medium in which measurement is performed (e.g. air, liquid). After one time constant (τ) thermistor presents 63.2% of new temperature value, measurement after 5 τ is considered sufficiently accurate.

Figure 3 presents the change of temperature indicated by thermistor in three situations:

- time constant = 1 s – for sensor only, i.e. for thermistor without encasement;

- time constant = 2 s – for complete probe, i.e. thermistor encased in PVC tube, during measurement in liquid;
- time constant = 2 s – for complete probe, i.e. thermistor encased in PVC tube, during measurement in still air.

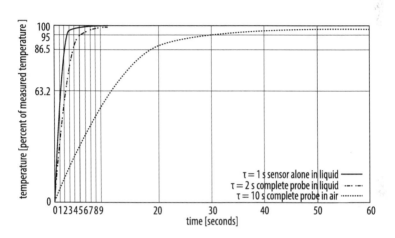

Figure 3. Measurement duration

Source: Study by Jacek Majkowski.

The horizontal axis represents time, where 0 stands for beginning of measurement. The vertical axis represents temperature, where 0 stands for initial thermistor temperature just before the measurement, while 100% is the new temperature value of thermistor. For a better understanding let us consider an example: after a long walk mountain rescuers take out of their backpack a probe, whose temperature is 5°C, and start measurement of patient's body, whose temperature is 35°C. The difference between initial temperature of the thermistor and its new temperature is 30°C. For 2 s time constant of a sensor, 2 s is time after which 63.2% of change of temperature is achieved (or 0.632 × 30°C = 19°C). Adding the initial temperature of probe (5°C) yields 24°C temperature indication. After 5 time constants, i.e. 10 s, 5°C + 0.994 × 30°C = 34.4°C is achieved, what is a satisfactory actual temperature approximation.

Attention: for 10 s time constant of a probe, i.e. in still air, e.g. in a situation when there is no direct contact between a sensor in an ear canal and tympanic membrane, measurement duration will be significantly prolonged – to at least 50 s. It is a consequence of a fact that thermal equilibrium with tympanic membrane must be achieved both by sensor as well as by air, which accepts the temperature of environment.

How to measure temperature well

Firstly, it must be remembered that thermometer demonstrates the temperature of the sensor – it is our role to make sure that during measurement the temperature of sensor is the same as of the object of measurement. That is why precise placement as well as selection of appropriate method are crucial. It should be noted here that infra-red, non-contact thermometers for use in ear canal measure the temperature of ear canal only and not the tympanic membrane (whose temperature approximates the brain temperature – core temperature). Even though in most situations the temperatures are similar, in hypothermia they differ significantly.

Contact methods (e.g. measurement with thermistor probe) necessitate appropriately long measurement time before thermic equilibrium between sensor and body measured is achieved. The result remains unstable until the sensor assumes the temperature of the measured body.

Place of measurement

Superficial temperature of human body differs in distribution of values and may not constitute a qualification criterium for extracorporeal treatment (Figure 4). Undertaking body temperature measurement in order to confirm hypothermia, the personnel is obliged to measure core temperature. Core temperature measurement should be understood as measurement in lower 1/3 of oesophagus, in urinary bladder, rectum or on tympanic membrane.

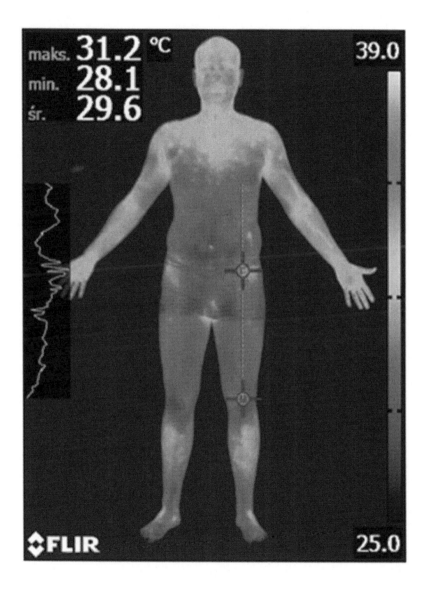

Figure 4. Distribution of cutaneous temperature measured with thermal imaging camera

Source: From collection of Department of Battlefield Medicine, Military Institute of Medicine, Warsaw, Poland.

5

Prehospital Management of Hypothermia

Paweł Podsiadło

Polish Medical Air Rescue, Kielce branch, Polish Society of Mountain Medicine and Rescue

Patient assessment

A patient suspected of hypothermia requires special treatment. Evaluation of hypothermia severity and prevention of iatrogenic cardiac arrest are crucial. The gold standard measurement for core temperature is measurement in lower 1/3 of oesophagus, what can be problematic in conscious patients retaining vomiting reflex [1]. Methods of temperature measurement have been described in Chapter 4 of this book.

If a prehospital rescue team possess no appropriate thermometer an approximate assessment should be performed with Swiss Staging System devised for this purpose [2] – Table 1.

The original Swiss classification published in 2003 has been updated [2].

Table 1. Update Swiss Staging System

Stage	Clinical Findings	Core temperature (if available)
Hypothermia I (mild) HT I	Conscious; shivering	35–32°C
Hypothermia II (moderate) HT II	Impaired consciousness; may or may not be shivering	< 32–28°C
Hypothermia III (severe) HT III	Unconscious; vital signs present	< 28°C
Hypothermia IV (severe) HT IV	Apparent death; Vital signs absent	Variable

Source: Own compiled upon Brown D.J.A. *Hypothermia*. In: Tintinalli J.E. ed. *Emergency Medicine*. 8ᵗʰ ed. McGraw Hill, New York 2015: 1357–1365 [2].

Searching for presence of breath and pulse should take at least 1 minute
[3]. Difficulties in diagnosis result from breath becoming significantly slow
and shallow, and from bradycardia with low systemic blood pressure. Wrong
diagnosis of cardiac arrest and erroneous commencement of CPR may lead
to ventricular fibrillation (VF) [4]. ECG displayed on monitor may be helpful
– VF or asystole require instant commencement of resuscitation. Presence
of organised rhythm necessitates verification of spontaneous circulation.
In absence of palpable pulse, capnography (distinctive "wavy" capnogram
suggests presence of circulation) or ultrasonography may be used [1].

Freezing of body tissues makes chest compressions impossible, evident fatal injuries such as decapitation, major crush injuries of the trunk
etc. and unequivocal asphyxiation preceding hypothermia (burial, drowning in warm water) are situations where no indications for resuscitation
exist. In all other patients in whom hypothermia occurred with patent
airways, regardless of body temperature, the rule "nobody is dead until
warm and dead" should be applied [1, 3].

Management of basic body functions

Circulatory system

In the natural course of cooling of the heart, cardiac arrest occurs in asystole [4]. Hypothermic heart, however, is very prone to VF as a result of
various, even very slight stimuli: mechanical (rough transportation, ambulation, resuscitation), changes in pH (excessively aggressive ventilation),
changes of temperature (afterdrop). It is most likely a result of non-uni-
form prolongation of action potential in various areas of myocardium (re-
fraction dispersion) and forming of looped impulse circuit (reentry) [4, 5].
Ventricular fibrillation in severe hypothermia is resistant to pharmacotherapy and electric defibrillation. Three shocks are accepted in core temperature < 30°C, further shocks should be delivered after rewarming of the
patient above 30°C [3, 4]. Cases of reverting to sinus rhythm even in 24°C
have been reported, yet such cases remain exceptional [6].

Bradycardia in hypothermia is similarly resistant to treatment. Pharmacotherapy proves inefficient, electric stimulation requires high energy

and increases risk of VF [4]. As long as bradycardia remains adequate for reduced metabolic demands of hypothermic organism, no interventions beyond rewarming should be undertaken.

The administered drugs are not metabolised at sufficient rate in low body temperature what may lead to their accumulated effect after rewarming. The most efficient method of treatment of heart arrhythmias in hypothermia is rewarming of the patient [3].

During CPR, the method and frequency of chest compressions are the same as in patients in normothermia. If prolonged resuscitation is expected, it is optimal to implement mechanical chest compressions device [1, 3].

Respiratory system

Metabolic rate and oxygen demand drop with decrease of body temperature. The respiratory system responds adequately by slowed and shallow breathing. If however shivering occurs, demand for oxygen increases significantly, what should be kept in mind when ventilating the patient [7, 8]. The principles and methods of airway management in hypothermia are described in Chapter 7 of this book.

In patients breathing spontaneously in mild or moderate hypothermia, a moderate hypercapnia (about 30–35 mmHg) is likely. Even lower values of $PaCO_2$ should be expected in severe hypothermia. The reasons for this are: slowing of metabolic rate, and increased solubility of carbon dioxide in plasma (see: Chapter 1). Hypocapnia in spontaneously breathing patient can be interpreted as {a sign of} adaptation to reduced body temperature. Thus technique of mechanical ventilation should be adjusted to reduced metabolic rate. In order to achieve this, reduction of rate of respirations even by half in comparison to normothermia may be necessary [1]. When establishing ventilation parameters in hypothermia, values of end-tidal carbon dioxide (EtCO$_2$) should not be used as a strict guideline. Physical properties of CO_2 in low temperatures, disorders of ventilation and pulmonary perfusion, variable lungs compliance, as well as unpredictable individual factors may cause end-tidal carbon dioxide values to differ significantly from arterial levels. Maintaining "ventilation stability" is important, together with avoidance of sudden changes in rate and volume of respirations – all modification to the parameters should be introduced gradually.

In perfect conditions, the oxygen administered to the patient should be warmed to 40°C and humidified [8]. Unfortunately, transport ventilators are usually unable to meet these requirements, and devices able to operate in the outdoors are not widely available. Breathing filters partially serve a purpose of heat and moisture exchangers.

Interruption of exposure to cold

Stopping further cooling of patient's body may present a serious challenge, depending on site of incident and meteorological conditions. Loss of heat is prompted by contact with cold surface, wet clothing and wind. Transporting the patient to warm environment, removal of wet clothing, and placing the patient in warm sleeping bag constitute optimal measures. Thermic insulation of head is of great importance as the area is characterised by major heat loss. Particular caution is necessary when undressing the patient in severe hypothermia; cutting the clothing, as it is practiced with traumatic patients, seems safer [1, 3, 10]. Movement of extremities leads to risk of forcing the cold blood into the trunk and, as a consequence, occurrence of VF as a result of sudden afterdrop. In unfavourable conditions, in cold interior, and especially during exposure to wind, leaving the wet clothes and wrapping the patient in several insulating layers (sleeping bags, blankets, plastic wrap)most likely poses smaller risk of further cooling of the body than removal of clothing and exposure to external conditions [8].

Achieving homeostasis equilibrium

Pathophysiology of hypothermia implies two crucial deficits necessitating intervention in prehospital phase of treatment.

The first one is hypoglycaemia which occurs in slow cooling of the body with prolonged shivering (muscular contractions consume major amounts of glucose) [4]. In some patients this co-occurs with hypoglycaemia induced by alcohol consumption. During rewarming the patient may present shivering anew, what necessitates repeated glucose supplementation. Another obstacle may be low ambient temperature during blood glucose testing (slowing of enzymatic reaction on test strip). Glucometer itself is standardised to operate in specific range of temperatures, usually above 0°C. If glucose measurement is not possible, glucose should be administered "on spec."

The phenomenon of "cold diuresis" is the reason for hypovolaemia in hypothermic patients. Fluid replacement in hypothermia is associated with particular precautions. Cold intravenous fluids administration precipitates further decrease in patient's core temperature [4, 9]. Concept of "warmed infusion" should denote fluid entering the vein, not merely warmth of infusion container. In a cold interior (heated interior of an ambulance in wintertime is between 10–20°C maximum) heat loss during the fluid flow through non-insulated tube may result in actual fluid administered to the vein possessing the temperature of the surrounding air [11]. The solution to the problem, besides thermal insulation of the container and tubing, are fluid heating devices installed onto tubing or wounding of tubing onto heating pad. When choosing i.v. infusion it should be kept in mind that colloids may disturb blood coagulation process (already impaired by hypothermia) and that hydroxyethyl starch (HES) infusions must not be heated above 25°C. Dextran infusions may cause polymerisation of cryofibrinogen and unwanted increase in blood viscosity [4]. Crystalloids appear as safe, excluding those with lactates content (as liver during hypothermia is unable to efficiently metabolise them) [1]. Fast infusions of large volumes should be avoided on grounds of lowered heart contractility and risk of pulmonary oedema.

Commencement of rewarming

Rewarming, as treatment of hypothermia cause, should be commenced as early as it is possible, already on the site of incident or during transportation [1, 3, 9]. Shivering in hypothermic patient is a physiological mechanism of thermogenesis. Shivering, however, increases demand for oxygen and carbohydrates. Conscious patient should thus be given warm, sweet drinks, the unconscious one should have i.v. infusion of glucose started. In severe hypothermia no shivering occurs and patient must be rewarmed using active methods. The first response medical teams have at their disposal: chemical heating pads exothermic reaction of supersaturated solution), electric blankets with independent energy source, i.v. infusions warmed in heater and {variety of} improvised methods. The heat source must not have a direct contact with skin (risk of burns), and its temperature should not exceed 45°C [12]. Heating pads should be placed in the armpits, on chest and on back. Limbs should not be warmed, but also need not be insulated from the heat source. IMPORTANT – contact with external heat source and administration of certain drugs, e.g. opioid analgesics, may halt shivering – in such situations active rewarming should be continued [1, 8]. Rewarming the patient on site should not delay commencement of transport to hospital, particularly in severe hypothermia with circulatory instability.

Monitoring

Because of high risk of cardiac arrest, hypothermic patient should be attentively monitored on the way to hospital. Cool skin possesses increased impedance, what may make obtaining ECG reading on monitor difficult. Adhesive electrodes or improvised needle electrodes (thin needles placed shallow the skin of the patient and passing through electrodes in place of cable connection) may enable acceptable ECG reading [13]. Constriction of peripheral vessels caused by cold often renders oxygen saturation reading with pulse oximeter impossible. For this reason it seems justified to increase concentration of oxygen in air inhaled by the patient so as to prevent hypoxia, particularly in shivering [3, 8]. Capnometry, as a method little affected by temperature, is an useful indicator of presence of spontaneous circulation.

Transportation

Decisions concerning the form of evacuation and transportation of patient depend on stage of hypothermia and local conditions on site of accident. The general rule is to use passive transportation of the patient in supine position, what allows to decrease afterdrop.

Patient in mild hypothermia (HT 1) who is conscious and shivering can be allowed to walk if it quickens the arrival in safe place. Ambulation and walk should be preceded by half an hour of passive rewarming (shivering with good thermal insulation) and administering of warm, sweet drink [1, 9]. Patients in advanced stages of hypothermia must be transported in supine position of the body. Reduced cardiac output, hypovolaemia and hypotonia may cause loss of consciousness or even cardiac arrest after an attempt of ambulation (rescue collapse) [1, 9, 10]. Prohibition of ambulation concerns all phases of patient transportation, including the process the retrieving the patient from water, under snow in avalanche etc. All manoeuvres related to moving the patient must be particularly cautious on account of danger of triggering VF. Resuscitation during the evacuation in demanding terrain may be indispensable, moments when continuation of CPR become dangerous or impossible may occur. Brief pauses in resuscitation are acceptable in order to advance evacuation, on grounds of reduced metabolic rate and protective action of cold onto brain [14]. It is however a choice of "lesser evil", which can be avoided by use of mechanical chest compression devices. Appropriately early information about search for a hypothermic patient allows delivery of such a device onto site of incident.

Transport destination for patients with unstable circulation or in cardiac arrest (HT 3 and HT 4) is a hospital with extracorporeal rewarming (ECMO, CPB) capacity. It is acceptable, in certain situations, to transport the patient to such facility directly, bypassing emergency ward. The rules for qualification for extracorporeal rewarming have been described in Chapter 19.

References

1. Zafren K., Giesbrecht G.G., Danzl D.F. et al. *Wilderness Medical Society Practice Guidelines for the Out-of-Hospital Evaluation and Treatment of Accidental Hypothermia.* Wilderness Environ. Med. 2014; 25: 425–445.
2. Brown D.J.A. *Hypothermia.* In: Tintinalli J.E. ed. *Emergency Medicine.* 8th ed. McGraw Hill, New York 2015: 1357–1365.
3. Soar J., Perkins G.D., Abbas G. et al. *European Resuscitation Council Guidelines for Resuscitation 2010 Section 8. Cardiac arrest in special circumstances: Electrolyte abnormalities, poisoning, drowning, accidental hypothermia, hyperthermia, asthma, anaphylaxis, cardiac surgery, trauma, pregnancy, electrocution.* Resuscitation 2010; 81: 1400–1433.

4. Mallet M.L. *Pathophysiology of accidental hypothermia*. Q. J. Med. 2002; 95: 775–785.

5. Southwick F.S., Dalglish P.H. Jr. *Recovery after prolonged asystolic cardiac arrest in profound hypothermia*. JAMA 1980; 243: 1250–1253.

6. Clift J., Munro-Davies L. *Is defibrillation effective in accidental severe hypothermia in adults?* Emerg. Med. J. 2007; 24: 50–51.

7. Giesbrecht G.G., Goheen M.S.L., Johnston C.E. et al. *Inhibition of shivering increases core temperature afterdrop and attenuates rewarming in hypothermic humans*. J. Appl. Physiol. 1997; 83: 1630–1634.

8. Danzl D.F., Lloyd E.L. *Treatment of accidental hypothermia*. W: *Medical Aspects of Harsh Environments*, vol. 1. Borden Institute Walter Reed Army Medical Center, Washington, DC 2001.

9. Brown D., Brugger H., Boyd J. et al. *Accidental hypothermia. Current concepts*. N. Engl. J. Med. 2012; 367: 1930–1938.

10. Giesbrecht G.G. *Prehospital treatment of hypothermia*. Wilderness Environ. Med. 2001; 12: 24–31.

11. Handrigan M.T., Wright R.O., Becker B.M. et al. *Factors and methodology in achieving ideal delivery temperatures for intravenous and lavage fluid in hypothermia*. Am. J. Emerg. Med. 1997; 15: 350–353.

12. Mulcahy A., Watts M. *Accidental hypothermia: an evidence-based approach*. Emerg. Med. Practice 2009; 11(1): 1–23

13. Weinberg A.D. *Hypothermia*. Ann. Emerg. Med. 1993; 22(Pt 2): 370–377.

14. Gordon L., Paal P., Ellerton J.A. et al. *Delayed and intermittent CPR for severe accidental Hypothermia*. Resuscitation 2015; 90: 46–49.

6

Thermal Insulation

Sylweriusz Kosiński[1,2,3], Tomasz Sanak[1,4,5]

[1] "Heat for Life" Foundation, Cracow, Poland
[2] Department of Anaesthesiology and Intensive Care, Pulmonary Hospital, Zakopane, Poland
[3] Tatra Mountain Rescue Service, Zakopane
[4] Department of Disaster Medicine and Emergency Care, Jagiellonian University Collegium Medicum, Cracow, Poland
[5] Department of Battlefield Medicine, Military Institute of Medicine, Warsaw, Poland

Maintaining homeothermy (stable body temperature) requires equilibrium between heat generated by the organism and dissipated to the environment [1]. Each living cell of the body produces heat as a side-effect of metabolic processes. Apart from this "basic" production, heat is generated also during physical effort, and its amount is proportional to the intensity of the activity. It is worth noting that certain amount of thermic energy may be "absorbed" from the outside via the same pathways it is lost. On a sunny winter day, when ambient temperature is 0–5°C, we may do without warm clothing as we absorb significant amount of solar radiation. In a cold room we stand close to a hot radiator, and desiring to get warmer faster, we put our back close to it. In moments of danger we have one more heat generation method at our disposal – shivering (see: Chapter 1).

Intensity of metabolic processes, including heat generation, depends on many factors: weight, sex, age, physical activity, ambient temperature, type of cover/clothing. In emergency care, the disorders reducing metabolic rate may be of additional importance, in particular: severe injuries, exhaustion – understood as deficit of energy substrates, and influence of medications.

Mechanisms of heat loss (conduction, convection, radiation and evaporation) have been described in Chapters 1 and 3. As human being loses about 90% of heat through skin, the prevention of thermic imbalance should focus on body surface insulation. Are we able to stop the processes of heat transferral to the surroundings entirely? Unfortunately not. Yet we can minimise them to such an extent so as to compensate even a severely limited production. Of course, in extreme cases the balance may be "tipped" by heat delivery, but this chapter aims to concentrate on means to prevent heat loss, i.e. thermal insulation.

First of all, let us use an example to illustrate the pathways of heat loss and counteraction measure. Let us compare streams of heat leaving the organism in two places: vicinity of Supraśl (Poland) and area of Spitsbergen (Norway) [2, 3] – Table 1.

Table 1. Heat exchange between human organism and the environment in different climate zones

Place	Convection W/m²	Evaporation W/m²	Radiation W/m²	Respiration W/m²	Total W/m²
Supraśl	−32.4	−23.7	−17.3	−5.5	−78.9
Spitsbergen	−249.8	−79.7	−38.1	−21.4	−389

Source: Own compiled upon: Krawczyk B., Błażejczyk K. *Heat Balance of the Human Body in the Urban Area (on the example of Supraśl)*. Acta Univ. Lodz. 1998; 3: 559–565 [2]; Dubicka M., Sikora S., Migała K. *Heat Balance of the Human Organism on Example of SW Spitsbergen (Bilans cieplny organizmu człowieka w warunkach polarnych na przykładzie SW Spitsbergenu)*. XV Ogólnopolskie Seminarium Meteorologii i Klimatologii Polarnej, Gdańsk 2005 [3].

In both places the studied subjects were clad in manner appropriate to climate conditions – in vicinity of Supraśl in cotton tracksuit (summer), in Arctic region in polar outfit (winter), in both situations the studied subjects undertook merely a light physical effort (slow walk). What does the comparison reveal? First, in cold environment, despite proper clothing and physical activity, we lose a vast amount of heat (over four times more than basic metabolic rate). Secondly, in both environments the dominating heat loss process is convection, in cold environment it is eight times greater than in the warm one. Thirdly, radiation in clothed people constitutes, surprisingly, only 20% of total heat loss in warm surroundings and about 10% in the cold.

What conclusions can be drawn for the medical professionals? Firstly, our efforts should concentrate on stopping the convective heat flux. Secondly, radiation is a less vital problem than commonly believed, and to reduce the loss by this process reflective covers are not necessary. Thirdly, in the face of such sizeable potential heat loss every condition which halts metabolic heat generation and/or disables movement of the body (e.g. injury, loss of consciousness) lead to hypothermia on short notice.

It should be remarked that in the comparison presented above conduction was not mentioned. The area of human feet is too small and usually to well insulated so as to constitute a significant heat loss pathway. The situation may radically change when sitting, and even more in horizontal position of the body. In studies conducted in operating theatre it was noticed that flux of heat transmitted to a well conducting bed of 25°C is as high as 120 W/m^2 [4]. Considering the fact that patients we are dealing with are very often in supine position, and surface they are placed upon may be cooler, insulation of the back of the body should be particularly observed.

In what way, thus, optimal product for thermic insulation of the patients should be designed and used? In many studies the term "active thermic insulation" is used, without clarifying what are its components. In most works multilayered cover is mentioned, which in practice is used rarely. In many instances improvised solutions are recommended, whose efficacy is hard to predict. Hence, it is worthwhile to approach the problem in a methodical manner.

The vacuum is the best insulator. In lack of vacuum a tight layer of still air serves the same purpose. This is the principle behind functionality of layered clothing – several layers of air between several layers of fabric usually ensure thermal comfort. In contemporary garments the manufacturers have gone a step further – by assigning specific functions to particular layers. The first layer (closest to the body) serves primarily to evacuate moisture. The last layer (the most external) is supposed to protect from wind and moisture. The middle layer provides actual thermic insulation. It is usually composed of thick and light fabric (e.g. polar fleece), with countless micro-pockets of air. The basic condition for efficacy of such clothing is tightness – the external (wind and waterproof) layer seals the system and traps the air inside. Any "draughts" affecting stability of air layers ruin the whole concept and enable convective heat loss. Apart from maintenance of tightness, the protection against moisture is another crucial task. Water penetrating between layers (e.g. rain, sweat), fills all air spaces of fabrics, reduces their protection efficacy and causes increased loss by evaporation and conduction. By translating these reasonings onto the language of emergency care we obtain the following guidelines:

- the fabrics used for thermal insulation must be dry and ensure tightness;
- there must be some free space between layers;
- it is optimal if one of the layers is composed of thick, light, "pneumatic" fabric such as: polar fleece, thick wool, natural or artificial down, etc.;
- if possible, hydrophilic (i.e. moisture absorbing) fabrics, such as cotton, should be avoided;
- external layer, protecting from wind and moisture, is particularly important during rescue efforts in open spaces;
- typical, improvised layered cover is of little practicality – the price for thickness is difficulty in access to the patient;
- systemic solutions are the best ones, e.g. sleeping bags; they are designed with horizontal position of the body in mind (good insulation from the ground) and manufactured from appropriate materials; access to the patient is quick when needed.

Insulation required index (IREQ) states to what degree given fabric protects from the cold. It is presented in thermal resistance units – clo (1 clo = 0.155 m^2K/W). Undressed person has clo = 0, typical office garment in neutral conditions has clo = 1, arctic outfit has about 4 clo. The best sleeping bags used in high altitude climbing have up to 10 clo. Generally speaking, clo depends on fabric thickness (about 1.3–1.5 clo/cm) and external conditions. In multilayered clothing particular clo values can be summed in order to obtain approximate value for the entire protective cover.

Considering the external conditions and thermic qualities of the fabrics, one can create a thermal barrier in all circumstances. However, a problem remains: as for now no requirements concerning thermic insulation index were stated for emergency care in various conditions. It is practical to have at least three kits ready: summer, winter and transitional (spring, autumn) ones. It is good to include local conditions (average yearly temperatures for various seasons, wind speed, etc.) in calculations. Assuming that heat generation in patients equals their basic metabolic rate (70 W/m²) and our goal is to maintain thermal equilibrium during longer exposure without causing reflex vasoconstriction (so called "neutral clo"), the following general rules are proposed [1]:

- summer {insulation} kit (ambient temperature 15–20°C) – from 1.5 to 2 clo;
- transitional {insulation} kit (ambient temperature 5–15°C) – from 2 to 3 clo;
- winter {insulation} kit (ambient temperature –5–0°C) – from 3.5 to 4.5 clo;
- mountain {insulation} kit (ambient temperature –10 and below, sudden changes possibility, major conductive heat loss) – > 6 clo;
- strong wind reduces basic clothing insulation of most materials by about 30% – increase in cover must compensate this;
- reduced metabolic rate (severe trauma, exhaustion, confirmed/suspected hypothermia) – 0.5–1 clo should be added.

Example

First response medical team was called to a 45 years old man accidentally shot in abdomen during a walk. The patient is conscious, in shock, estimated time to arrive back to ambulance and afterwards to hospital is about 45 minutes. Ambient temperature is –5°C, strong wind is blowing. The head of the team estimates that thermal resistance of the cover will have to amount to about 5 clo. Dry clothing of the patient may be about 1–1.5 clo. Additional insulation should be provided by two or three woollen blankets and aluminium foil as the external layer.

In emergency care many further issues must be taken into consideration. Supine position, as we remarked before, forces conductive flux to the surface below. Simultaneously, compression of insulating fabrics {on the back of the patient} reduces their efficacy, often very substantially. Consequently, no stretcher, spine board, toboggan etc. should be placed directly on cold ground. After having transported the patient to the interior of ambulance (or any other safe, heated room) loss of heat by convection, conduction and respiration becomes significantly reduced. In such situation, if we keep the same thermal insulation as outside, some of the patients may start to sweat. As a result, increased loss by evaporation becomes likely (Table 1). Although members of first response teams have many, often more urgent actions to take, it is worthwhile – even "on the fly" – to check current condition of the patient and necessary thermal insulation at a given moment.

Another problem, which in prehospital phase may be crucial, is wet clothing on patient. In some algorithms it is recommended to instantly remove wet clothing and replace it with dry one. If an exchange of covers is to take place in safe zone (e.g. interior of an ambulance, inside of building or a tent) the rule is indisputable. The removal of clothing in cold environment at incident site, however, is controversial. Firstly, even wet clothes provide some amount of thermal insulation [7]. Hygrophobic fabrics, e.g. wool or synthetics, lose only a minor portion of their thermic properties. Secondly, anyone who has ever removed wet clothing from a patient (e.g. retrieved from icy water at air temperature of –10°C) is aware how time consuming and relatively complicated this action is, endangering both the patient and the rescuers with hypothermia. Thirdly, patients suspected of severe hypothermia should be carefully immobilised in supine position, if possible, without bending of major joints and sudden changes of body position. Clinical studies show that solution to this problem exists. It was shown that placing a waterproof cover (e.g. PVC wrap) on wet clothes of the patient, and subsequently providing the thermic insulation proper in form of several blankets is as efficient as removal of wet clothing and wrapping the patient in blankets [8, 9].

Mountain rescuers face further challenges, as their task is to provide thermal comfort to accident victims in extreme conditions and inaccessible locations. In such circumstances, besides the rules outlined above, additional and – as often happens – unconventional measures must be taken. Literally every square centimetre of the body must be insulated. For instance, skiing goggles not only protect the eyes from snow and ice, but also ensure thermic protection of the area. Respiratory heat loss may reach 1/3 of reduced metabolic production in cold environment (Table 1). Attempts must be made to limit this loss, by covering the mouth and nose with air-permeable fabric. If the patient is transported in toboggan on snow or ice, the back of the patient must be especially insulated. Atmospheric water (snow, rain, ice) which penetrates the external layer will have a tendency to gather in that area, reducing thermic properties of fabrics. The authors' experience shows that toboggan is best insulated with several layers of bubble wrap, which does not compress, does not absorb moisture and, additionally, provides mechanical comfort.

References

1. Cul A., Komorowicz T., Kupiec K. *Wymiana ciepła między człowiekiem a otoczeniem w mikroklimacie zimnym.* Czas. Tech. 2012; 17: 3–14.
2. Krawczyk B., Błażejczyk K. *Bilans cieplny człowieka w mieście na przykładzie Supraśla.* Acta Univ. Lodz. 1998; 3: 559–565.
3. Dubicka M., Sikora S., Migała K. *Bilans cieplny organizmu człowieka w warunkach polarnych na przykładzie SW Spitsbergenu.* XV Ogólnopolskie Seminarium Meteorologii i Klimatologii Polarnej, Gdańsk 2005.
4. Brauer A., Pacholik L., Perl T. et al. *Conductive heat exchange with a gel-coated circulating water mattress.* Anesth. Analg. 2004; 99: 1742–1746.
5. Ogulata R.T. *The effect of thermal insulation of clothing on human thermal comfort.* Fibres Text. East. Eur. 2007; 15: 67–72.
6. Henriksson O., Lundgren P., Kuklane K. et al. *Protection against cold in prehospital care – thermal insulation properties of blankets and rescue bags in different wind conditions.* Prehosp. Disaster Med. 2009; 24: 408–415.
7. Farnworth B., Dolhan P.A. *Heat loss through wet clothing insulation.* Defence Research Establishment, Ottawa 1983.
8. Henriksson O., Lundgren P., Kuklane K. et al. *Protection against cold in prehospital care: evaporative heat loss reduction by wet clothing removal or the addition of a vapor barrier – a thermal manikin study.* Prehosp. Disaster Med. 2012; 27: 53–58.
9. Thomassen Ø., Færevik H., Østerås Ø. et al. *Comparison of three different prehospital wrapping methods for preventing hypothermia – a crossover study in humans.* Scand. J. Trauma Resusc. Emerg. Med. 2011; 19: 41, doi: 10.1186/1757-7241-19-41.

7

Airway Management in Hypothermic Patients

Paweł Andruszkiewicz

2nd Clinic of Anaesthesiology and Intensive Care, Warsaw Medical University, Warsaw, Poland

Challenges

- Severe hypothermia causes grave disorders of respiratory system. Major decrease in body temperature causes disturbance of brain function, depression of respiratory centre in brain stem and impairment of defence reflexes of the airways [1].
- Severe stages of hypothermia are associated with increasing stiffness in skeletal muscles, what may cause difficulties in airways management [2]. The rescuer must be ready to face difficulties in tilting the head of the patient, limited degree to which mouth of the patient opens during insertion of oropharyngeal airway (OP), laryngeal mask airway (LMA) or laryngoscopy [3].
- Because of low incidence rate of hypothermia it cannot be unequivocally stated that hypothermic patients constitute a group of patients with expected difficulties in intubation, yet such statement may find grounds in pathophysiology of the disorder [2, 4].
- Hypothermic patients who are unconscious or in cardiac arrest constitute the group particularly threatened by aspiration of gastric contents. Passive movement of gastric contents to larynx (regurgitation) is a dangerous complication, which may lead both to mechanical obstruction of the airways as well as aspiration (chemical) pneumonitis [3]. In physiological conditions the stomach is emptied within 6 hours. Hypothermia may prolong this process.

- Stiffness of skeletal muscles increasing with hypothermia may cause decrease in chest compliance and lead to ventilation disorders. Reduced elasticity of chest walls may favour occurrence of atelectasis, disorders of ventilation/perfusion ratio (V/Q ratio) and pulmonary shunt [2, 5]. Lowered partial pressure of oxygen in blood may result.
- Settings where medical care is provided (prehospital setting, emergency ward) and competence of providers are important factors that determine scope of airway management.

Procedure

The goals of medical team dealing with patient in severe hypothermia are provision of adequate oxygenation and ventilation as well as protection from aspiration [3]. Definitive airway protection and implementation of efficient mechanical ventilation may present a major challenge for medical practitioners, particularly in prehospital setting. This is caused by time pressure, circumstances of CPR, varied experience of team members, as well as limited equipment. In such situations, proper and organised functioning of medical team is crucial.

Initial airway assessment

Assessment of airways for patency or obstruction is an integral part of evaluation of unconscious patient. On account of muscle stiffness this manoeuvre must be performed with special caution. European Resuscitation Council guidelines indicate necessity of verification of presence or absence of normal breathing after opening the airways. Recommendations indicate that search for vital signs in severe hypothermia should be prolonged to at least 1 minute before cardiac arrest is diagnosed [4].

Methods of airway management

In unconscious and in cardiac arrest patients advanced airway management is recommended. The definite and optimal method is endotracheal intubation. This technique protects the airways, facilitates mechanical ventilation and relieves a member of rescue team from constant involvement. Intubation should be, if possible, preceded by patient oxygenation [6, 7]. Careful endotracheal intubation should not be delayed if indications for the procedure occur. Although a minor risk of intubation triggering ventricular fibrillation exists, the benefits of correct ventilation and protection from aspiration prevail [4].

In patients breathing spontaneously an oxygen mask with reservoir bag (OMR) may be used, this enables administering oxygen concentrations up to 80% (oxygen flow: 10–15 L/min) [7]. It has not been confirmed that high flow of oxygen during oxygenation favours loss of heat by the patient.

In non-breathing patients oxygenation should be active, performed with manual resuscitator with reservoir bag (flow of oxygen 15 L/min) and PEEP valve attached. This method allows to reach oxygen concentrations exceeding 80%.

Verification of oxygen administration in pre-hospital setting is very limited on account of circulatory centralisation, what makes obtaining of plethysmographic reading and measurement of blood oxygen saturation practically impossible.

Repeated attempts of endotracheal tube (ETT) insertion without mechanical ventilation and chest compressions (in cardiac arrest) are unacceptable. The percentage of failures or difficulties in intubation can be significantly reduced by usage of many devices facilitating endotracheal tube insertion [3]. It appears that in pre-hospital and emergency ward settings videolaryngoscopes are particularly useful, which enable visualisation of laryngoscopy and tube manipulations on screen.

The risk of gastric contents aspiration necessitates choice of rapid sequence intubation (RSI) [8]. Application of pressure onto cricoid cartilage (Sellick manoeuvre) with force of 30 N was recommended in classical RSI algorithm. It was believed that this manoeuvre could occlude the oesophagus by compressing it between larynx and spinal column. Recent years brought questioning of this theory and emphasis on lateral displacement of oesophagus in relation to larynx and spine.

Confirmation of tube placement in trachea is indispensable after intubation attempt [3]. In prehospital setting and in limited diagnostic capabilities, auscultation of chest in mid-clavicular lines for symmetric vesicular sounds, and chest movements during mechanical ventilation are imperative. Capnography should also be used. In cardiac arrest and low cardiac output syndromes (LCOS), including severe hypothermia, analysis of end-tidal carbon dioxide is hindered (see Chapter 5). In such situations use of portable ultrasonography may be particularly helpful, as it is becoming more popular in emergency wards and prehospital rescue. Imaging of pleural "sliding" sign and diaphragm movement is a secondary method of confirmation of ETT placement [9].

Oxygenation and ventilation are priorities in non-breathing patient. Intubation is not a goal of rescue personnel. Insufficient experience and failed attempts to intubate should persuade the personnel to implement alternative but efficient methods of airways management.

The simplest solution useful in such situations is properly fitted oropharyngeal airway (OPA). The most popular advanced airway is laryngeal mask airway (LMA), laryngeal tube (LT), which additionally enables mechanical ventilation attachment. In patients with high risk of aspiration, use of the latest generation of laryngeal masks (supraglottic airway device – SAD 2) appears as particularly grounded. The devices are equipped with additional lumen for gastric tube placement. Use of SAD 2 reduces the risk of stomach insufflation and allows the use of higher peak pressure in the airways. It may be of special importance when performing simultaneous chest compressions and ventilation.

Alternative airway devices, such as Combitube, may also be useful in airway management. Their popularity is however limited. Proper airway management enables mechanical ventilation.

It is worth noting that on site of incident, in low ambient temperature, endotracheal tubes lose their elasticity and may have a tendency to bend. Increased stiffness necessitates use of higher pressure in sealing cuff what may result in mucous membrane damage. Pressure in the sealing cuff should be particularly monitored during rewarming of the patient.

Proper fixation of ETT in low temperatures may also prove problematic. Neither adhesive tapes nor professional fixation devices guarantee stable and secure position. It is thus recommended to verify the fixation frequently and practice additional, manual stabilisation of ETT during changes in patient position.

Summary

Airway assessment and management in severely hypothermic patients are compliant with general medical standards. In emergency care procedures, specific impact of low temperature onto organism of the patient must be taken into consideration.

References

1. Hayashi N. ed. *Brain hypothermia. Pathology, pharmacology and treatment of severe brain injury.* Springer-Verlag, Tokio 2000.
2. Witzmann F.A. *The regulation of body temperature w Medical Physiology. Principles for clinical medicine*, ed. 3. Wolters Kluwer, Lippincot Williams & Wilkins, 2009.
3. Walls R.M., Murphy M.F. *Mannual of emergency airway management*, ed. 4. Wolters Kluwer, Lippincot Williams & Wilkins, 2011.
4. Truhlár A., Deakinc C.D., Soar J. et al. *European Resuscitation Council Guidelines for Resuscitation 2015, Section 4. Cardiac arrest in special circumstances.* Resuscitation 2015; 95: 148–201.
5. Rodriguez-Roisin R., Roca J. *Mechanisms of hypoxemia.* W: Pinsky R.M., Brochard L., Hedenstierna G., Antonelli M. eds. *Applied Physiology in intensive care*, ed. 3. Springer, Heidelberg, New York, Dordrecht, London 2012.
6. Brugger H., Durrer B., Elsensohn F. et al. *Resuscitation of avalanche victims: Evidence-based guidelines of the international commission for mountain emergency medicine (ICAR MECOM) intended for physicians and other advanced life support personnel.* Resuscitation 2013; 84: 539–546.
7. Weingard S.D., Leviatan R.M. *Preoxygenation and prevention of desaturation during emergency airway management.* Ann. Emerg. Med. 2012; 59: 165–176.
8. El-Orbany M., Connolly L.A. *Rapid sequence induction and intubation current controversy.* Anaest. Analg. 2010; 110: 1318–1325.
9. Kristensen M.S. *Ultrasonography in the management of the airway.* Acta Anaesthesiol. Scand. 2011; 55: 1155–1173.

8

ECG in Hypothermia

Dorota Sobczyk

John Paul II Hospital, Cracow, Poland

Hypothermia is defined as a drop of core temperature (usually measured in oesophagus or rectum) below 35°C. Impact of hypothermia onto electrical conduction system of heart was first described in 1892. The first observations concerning changes in ECG of a patient in accidental hypothermia date back to 1938. Hypothermia is associated with presence of characteristic changes in ECG, depending on hypothermia stage.

Motion artefacts related to shivering and tremors are characteristic of mild hypothermia (Figure 1) together with sinus bradycardia resulting from compensatory stimulation of sympathetic nervous system.

Prolonged exposure to low temperature significantly impairs both electric as well as mechanic activity of the heart. As a result of catecholamines release, advanced stages of hypothermia are distinguished by decreased peripheral vascular resistance and noticeable drop in cardiac output. Prolonging of action potential duration and decrease in conduction velocity in conduction system of the heart are related to delay in activation/inactivation of cellular ionic (sodium, potassium and calcium) currents. Hypothermia causes prolonging of both depolarisation duration as well as repolarisation of sinus node cells. Decrease of body temperature below 32°C causes substantial reduction of conduction velocity. In such situation, serious sinus bradycardia develops, with PR and QT/QTc intervals prolongation as well as prolongations of P wave, QRS and T wave durations (Figure 2). There is a non-linear relationship between reduced heart rate and decrease in core temperature. Prolongation of QT/QTc

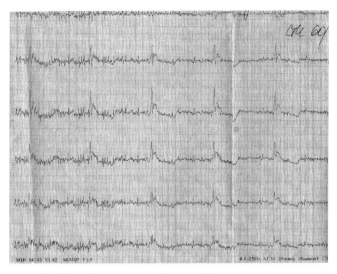

Figure 1. Sinus bradycardia, tremor artefacts visible

Source: Author's archive.

interval is caused both by delayed ventricular repolarisation and well as presence of so-called Osborn wave (J wave). In some patients, reduction of conduction velocity in atrio-ventricular node leads to development of conduction blocks.

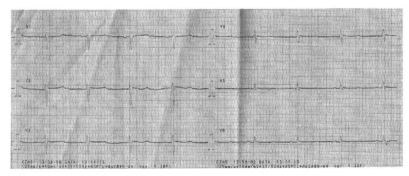

Figure 2. Sinus bradycardia, prolongation of PR and QT intervals as well as prolongation of QRS complex

Source: Author's archive.

Osborn wave (J wave) is certainly the most evident anomaly in ECG of hypothermic patients. Occurrence of the wave in hypothermic patients was first recorded in 1938 (Tomasjewski), but the full description of of the phenomenon was published in 1951 by J. Osborn (hence eponym). Osborn wave is a positive deflection appearing at junction between QRS complex and ST segment, resembling "camel hump" (Figure 3). It should be remembered that J wave is not a pathognomonic sign of hypothermia, and may occur also in hypercalcaemia, tricyclic antidepressants poisoning, and early repolarisation syndromes. In such disorders, presence of J wave is considered an prognostic of VF and sudden cardiac death (SCD) risk. In hypothermic patients no such relationship was established. J wave amplitude is inversely proportional to core temperature. No correlation between Osborn wave in ECG and electrolytes or pH levels has been proven. Osborn wave represents most probably an irregular depolarisation and repolarisation of myocardium. Osborn wave develops when core temperature falls below 32°C, and it occurs in up to 80% of patients with core temperature below 30°C.

Abnormalities to ST-T complex (elevation or depression of ST segment, flattening or inversion of T wave), which can imitate abnormalities in acute coronary syndromes, are directly related to acidosis and myocardium ischaemia. Abnormalities of T waves depend on hypothermia severity, and are inversely proportional to J wave amplitude.

Atrial extrasystoles and atrial arrhythmias are observed in core temperature below 29°C. Atrial fibrillation (typically with low ventricular rate) manifests itself in 50–60% of patients in moderate hypothermia (Figure 4). Occurrence of fast ventricular response during AF (atypical for hypothermia) is always caused by some additional disorder, such as hypovolaemia, sepsis or hypokalaemia. AF usually reverts to sinus rhythm during gradual rewarming or directly after achieving normothermia. No relationship between occurrence of AF and increased fatality in hypothermia was established. In such cases, possibility of mesenteric artery embolism must always be taken into consideration. Routine administration of anticoagulants is not recommended in expected fast arrhythmia reversal and on account of risk of hypothermia-related coagulopathy.

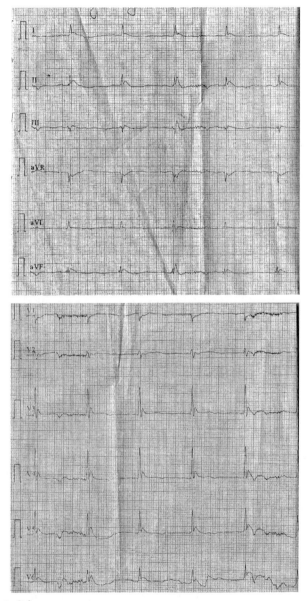

Figure 3. Osborn wave

Source: Author's archive.

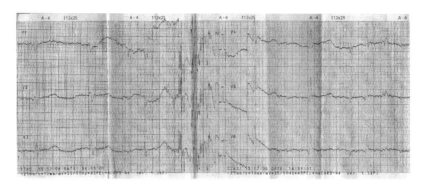

Figure 4. Atrial fibrillation with slow ventricular response

Source: Author's archive.

Further aggravation of hypothermia (core temperature below 2°C) is associated with risk of junctional rhythm and recursive arrhythmias. Differentiation between slow junctional rhythm and actual sinus bradycardia is usually difficult, particularly in presence of tremor artefacts. Patients in severe hypothermia are particularly at risk of ventricular fibrillation. Asystole occurs after decrease of core temperature below 26°C.

References

1. Brown D.J., Brugger H., Boyd J. et al. *Accidental hypothermia*. N. Engl. J. Med. 2012; 367: 1930–1938.
2. Kosinski S., Darocha T., Galazkowski R. et al. *Accidental hypothermia in Poland – estimation of prevalence, diagnostic methods and treatment*. Scand. J. Trauma Resusc. Emerg. Med. 2015; 23(1): 13.
3. Darocha T., Kosinski S., Jarosz A. et al. *Severe Accidental Hypothermia Center*. Eur. J. Emerg. Med. 2015; 22(4): 288–291.
4. Zafren K., Danzl D.F., Brugger H. et al. *Wilderness Medical Society Practice Guidelines for the Out-of-Hospital Evaluation and Treatment of Accidental Hypothermia*. Wilderness Environ. Med. 2014; 25(4): 425–445.
5. Doshi H.H., Giudici M.C. *The EKG in hypothermia and hyperthermia*. J. Electrocardiol. 2014; 48(2): 203–209 (http://dx.doi.org/10.1016/k.electrocard.2014.12.001; accessed: 19.10.2015).
6. Surawicz B., Childers R., Deal B.J. et al. *AHA/ACCF/HRS recommendations for the standardization and interpretation of the electrocardiogram: part III: intraven-*

tricular conduction disturbances. A scientific statement from the American Heart Association Electrocardiography and Arrhythmias Committee, Council on Clinical Cardiology; the American College of Cardiology Foundation; and the Heart Rhythm Society. Endorsed by the International Society for Computerized Electrocardiology. J. Am. Coll. Cardiol. 2009; 53(11): 976–981.

7. Rautaharju P.M., Surawicz B., Gettes L.S. et al. *AHA/ACCF/HRS recommendations for the standardization and interpretation of the electrocardiogram: part IV: the ST segment, T and U waves, and the QT interval. A scientific statement from the American Heart Association Electrocardiography and Arrhythmias Committee, Council on Clinical Cardiology; the American College of Cardiology Foundation; and the Heart Rhythm Society. Endorsed by the International Society for Computerized Electrocardiology.* J. Am. Coll. Cardiol. 2009; 53(11): 982–991.

8. Soar J., Perkins G.D., Abbas G. et al. *European Resuscitation Council Guidelines for Resuscitation 2010. Section 8. Cardiac arrest in special circumstances: Electrolyte abnormalities, poisoning, accidental hypothermia, hyperthermia, asthma, anaphylaxis, cardiac surgery, trauma, pregnancy, electrocution.* Resuscitation 2010; 81: 1400–1433.

9. Higuchi S., Takahashi T., Kabeya Y. *J waves in accidental hypothermia – body temperature and its clinical implications.* Circ. J. 2014; 78: 128–134.

10. Lebiedz P., Meiners J., Samol A. *Electrocardiographic changes during therapeutic hypothermia.* Resuscitation 2012; 83: 602–606.

11. Khan J.N., Prasad N., Glancy J.M. *QTc prolongation during therapeutic hypothermia: are we giving it the attention it deserves?* Europace 2010; 12: 266–270.

12. Osborn J.J. *Experimental hypothermia: respiratory and blood pH changes in relation to cardiac function.* Am. J. Physiol. 1953; 175: 389–398.

13. De Souza D., Perez Riera A.R., Bombing M.T. et al. *Electrocardiographic changes by accidental hypothermia in an urban and tropical region.* J. Electrocardiol. 2007; 40: 47–52.

14. Rolfast C.L., Lust E.J., de Cock C.C. *Electrocardiographic changes in therapeutic hypothermia.* Crit. Care 2012; 16: R100.

15. Omar H.R., Camporesi E.M. *The correlation between the amplitude of Osborn wave and core body temperature.* Eur. Heart J. Acute Cardiovasc. Care 2014. Epub ahead of print.

16. Yan G.X., Antzelevitch C. *Cellular basis for the electrocardiographic J wave.* Circulation 1996; 93: 372–379.

9

Hypothermia as a Reversible Cause of Cardiac Arrest

Piotr Mazur[1], Sylweriusz Kosiński[3,4,5], Tomasz Darocha[2,3]

[1] Institute of Cardiology, Jagiellonian University Collegium Medicum; John Paul II Hospital, Cracow, Poland
[2] Severe Hypothermia Treatment Centre, Department of Anaesthesiology and Intensive Care, John Paul II Hospital, Cracow, Poland
[3] "Heat for Life" Foundation, Cracow, Poland
[4] Department of Anaesthesiology and Intensive Care, Pulmonary Hospital, Zakopane, Poland
[5] Tatra Mountain Rescue Service, Zakopane, Poland

Hypothermia, defined as unintended drop in core temperature < 35°C, is one of cardiac arrest causes which have been proven to be reversible. Hypothermia is one of "Hs" in universally accepted "4Hs + 4Ts" algorithm. Hypothermia however has one major advantage over the remaining "Hs" and all "Ts." Not only when early diagnosed and appropriately treated it may change the outcome of resuscitation, but it additionally increases chances of both survival as well as avoidance of ischaemic encephalopathy. Each 1°C of drop of body temperature below norm causes decrease of brain metabolism by 6–10% [1]. Hypothermia affects almost all cell damage mechanisms caused by hypoxia, by preventing their activation or interrupting them on early stage of apoptosis [2]. Intended, induced and controlled hypothermia is increasingly more often used in all these situations in which neuroprotective effect is desired. In emergency care the rule "No one is dead until warm and dead" exists. This phrase, however, proves right under a condition: hypothermia may show its protective action only if it occurs before cardiac arrest. Secondary hypothermia, which develops e.g. during resuscitation in cold environment, not only does not provide neuroprotection, but may be an obstacle in attempts to restore circulation. If however cardiac arrest occurs during cooling of the body or is a direct effect of it, the neurological prognosis is good – provided of course that circulation is restored. The longest reported resuscitation of hypothermic patient resulting in return of spontaneous circulation, restoring of consciousness and full neurological capabilities, endured for over 6.5 hours [3]. This and other reported cases prove that hypothermia may the most optimistic of "4Hs and 4Ts."

Unfortunately, it happens in practice that all hopes related to hypothermia become ruined. The usual reason for this is lack of diagnostic sensitivity. Hypothermia is one of the least frequent reversible causes of cardiac arrest listed in "4Hs and 4Ts." What is partially understandable, more attention is given to hypoxia, hypovolaemia or thromboembolisms, while hypothermia is considered a mostly theoretical issue. It also happens that overcome with first impression we consider a hypothermic patient to be dead, after only a superficial, imprecise examination and no resuscitation attempt is made. Vital signs are very hard to observe [4]. Skin is very cold, in some cases frost and ice may gather in skin inflections in peripheral parts of limbs. External tissues are stiff, and pulse palpation is hindered. It happens that the only method of verification of ongoing circulation is imaging myocardium contractions (usually very weak) by USG. Respirations are shallow and infrequent – in extreme cases 4–5 breaths per minute. Joints, particularly the peripheral ones, bend with difficulty. Pupils are usually broad and do not respond to light. The picture is completed by paleness and cyanosis (in peripheral body parts). As a result, even experienced members of medical staff may have serious doubts whether patient is in severe hypothermia or dead [5]. Further problems are associated with temperature measurement – clinical and practical aspects have been described in Chapter 4.

In cardiac arrest it is not possible to determine any of clinical signs listed in Swiss Staging System. Coldness of peripheral tissues is an extremely subjective type of examination, as the result depends on temperature of examiner's palms. Temperature measurement is not always possible and not always reliable (see Chapter 4). In many instances, only detailed medical history and/or circumstances of the incident may point to hypothermia. If such is the case, resuscitation should be commenced and continued at least until reliable temperature measurement is available.

When can we assume that patient cannot be helped and resuscitation is to no avail? According to Swiss Staging System the borderline between reversible hypothermia (HT 4) and irreversible one is freezing of tissues to a degree that compressing them is impossible [6], i.e. when areas usually soft to palpation become stiff, and do not yield when compressed. Unfortunately, this examination is subjective as well, and depends to a large extent on examiner's experience. The lowest survivable value of core temperature has not yet been established. Currently, the lowest temperature after which the patient has recovered with good neurological outcome was 13.7°C [7]. Yet the case of hypothermic boy found outdoors in vicinity of Kraków may lower the lowest survived temperature to 12°C! (not published). Longest total resuscitation with good outcomes – 65 years female, temperature 20.8°C. Asystole. Resuscitation was CPR (4 h 48 m) and ECLS (3 h 52 m). Total resuscitation time was 8 hours 40 minutes [8].

So, to rephrase it once again: if the circumstances of the incident suggest hypothermia, resuscitation should be commenced and continued at least until reliable temperature measurement is available. All doubts or dilemmas should be resolved with the greatest good of the patient in mind.

Resuscitation efforts should follow current guidelines of European Resuscitation Council. Modifications of the algorithm, as compared to normothermic patients, and special situations have been summarised in Table 1.

Resuscitation attempts may be futile if simultaneous intensive rewarming is not under way. In patients in cardiac arrest, extracorporeal rewarming methods are indicated, which provide the fastest rate of core temperature elevation, as well as circulatory and respiratory support [4, 6, 9].

Table 1. Modifications to PCR protocol in hypothermia

Phase	Actions
clinical assessment	Search for vital signs should take at least 1 minute. Simultaneous search for pulse and ECG rhythm analysis is recommended. Echocardiography, NIRS and Doppler ultrasound may be used to evaluate myocardium contractility. In any doubts, CPR should be commenced instantly.
start/termination of CPR	In prehospital settings, not starting the CPR in hypothermic patients is acceptable only when causes of cardiac are unequivocally: fatal injury, terminal illness, prolonged asphyxia or condition when chest compressions are unfeasible. In hospital, prior to decision to terminate CPR on a patient in severe hypothermia, a team of experiences physicians must be summoned in order to perform clinical evaluation.
airways management	Endotracheal intubation should not be delayed if indications exist. Although minor risk of triggering VF by intubation exists, the benefits of adequate ventilation and protection from aspiration prevail.
chest compressions	Hypothermia may cause stiffness of chest walls what may make ventilation and chest compressions difficult. Use of mechanical chest compression devices is recommended. If during prehospital phase maintaining of continuous CPR is impossible (e.g. during demanding transport), in core temperature < 28°C (or unknown) CPR should be carried out for 5 minutes intermitted by pauses ≤ 5 minutes. In patients with Tc < 20°C CPR carried out for 5 minutes and intermitted by pauses ≤ 10 minutes is acceptable [9].
pharmacotherapy	In hypothermia drug metabolism in is slowed, leading to potentially toxic plasma concentrations of any drugs given repeatedly. It recommended to withhold any drugs administration until patients Tc ≥ 30°C. Once 30°C has been reached, the intervals between drug doses should be doubled when compared with normothermia intervals (i.e. adrenalin should be given every 6—10 minutes). As normothermia is approached (over 35°C), standard drug protocols should be used. In hypothermia-induced cardiac arrest the efficacy of amiodarone is low.

treatment of arrhythmias	With decrease of core temperature, sinus bradycardia evolves into AF, followed by VF and eventually asystole. Arrhythmias other than VF tend to revert spontaneously as the core temperature increases, and usually do not require immediate treatment. Bradycardia may be physiological in severe hypothermia, and cardiac pacing is not indicated unless bradycardia associated with haemodynamic compromise persists after rewarming. In VF defibrillations should be given according to standard protocol. If the first shocks are ineffective, further shocks should be delayed until core temperature reaches $\geq 30°C$.
rewarming	CPR is not effective is the patient is not simultaneously rewarmed. All available active rewarming methods should be implemented, extracorporeal rewarming methods are however optimal.
transport	Patients in HT I and HT II with stable circulation should be transported to the nearest hospital. Patients in HT III and HT IV with circulatory instability (i.e. SBP < 90 mmHg, ventricular arrhythmia, Tc < 28°C) should be transported to medical center with extracorporeal life support (ECLS) capability, optimally ECMO.

Source: Own compilation upon Truhlář A., Deakinc C.D., Soar J. et al. *European Resuscitation Council Guidelines for Resuscitation 2015, Section 4. Cardiac arrest in special circumstances.* Resuscitation 2015; 95: 148–201 [4].

References

1. Hagerdal M., Harp J., Nilsson L. et al. *The effect of induced hypothermia upon oxygen consumption in the rat brain.* J. Neurochem. 1975; 24: 311–316.
2. Xu L., Yenari M.A., Steinberg G.K. et al. *Mild hypothermia reduces apoptosis of mouse neurons in vitro early in the cascade.* J. Cereb. Blood Flow Metab. 2002; 22: 21–28.
3. Lexow K. *Severe accidental hypothermia: survival after 6 hours 30 minutes of cardiopulmonary resuscitation.* Arctic Med. Res. 1991; 50(Suppl. 6): 112–114.
4. Truhlář A., Deakinc C.D., Soar J. et al. *European Resuscitation Council Guidelines for Resuscitation 2015, Section 4. Cardiac arrest in special circumstances.* Resuscitation 2015; 95: 148–201.
5. Brown D.J., Brugger H., Boyd J., *Accidental hypothermia.* N. Engl. J. Med. 2012; 367: 1930–1938.
6. Durrer B., Brugger H., Syme D., International Commission for Mountain Emergency M. *The medical on-site treatment of hypothermia: ICAR-MEDCOM recommendation.* High Alt. Med. Biol. 2003; 4: 99–103.
7. Gilbert M., Busund R., Skagseth A. et al. *Resuscitation from accidental hypothermia of 13.7 degrees C with circulatory arrest.* Lancet 2000; 355: 375–376.
8. Sepehripour A.H., Gupta S., Lall K.S. *When should cardiopulmonary bypass be used in the setting of severe hypothermic cardiac arrest?* Interact. Cardiovasc. Thorac. Surg. 2013; 17: 564–569.
9. Gordon L., Paal P., Ellerton J.A. et al. *Delayed and intermittent CPR for severe accidental hypothermia.* Resuscitation 2015; 90: 46–49.

10

The Role and Tasks of Polish Medical Air Rescue

Robert Gałązkowski

Department of Emergency Medical Services, Medical University, Warsaw, Poland
Polish Medical Air Rescue, Warsaw, Poland

Continuing advancement of medical science and advent of new techno-
logies have enabled efficient treatment of patients in severe hypothermia.
The efficacy of therapeutic process of these patients is possible thanks to
organisation of hypothermia treatment system, which encompasses both
prehospital as well in-hospital care phases. Emergency medical system,
which beside land ambulances includes also air rescue teams, provides
medical life-saving capability as well as translocation with intensive care
capacity to centres that ensure focused, specialised therapy.

Polish Medical Air Rescue, as a part of National Emergency Medical
System, so as to aid successfully developing program of treatment of severe hypothermia has undertaken organisational and educational actions
aiming at active participation of medical air rescue teams in saving hypothermic patients.

Medical air rescue teams possess equipment enabling direct invasive
blood pressure and core temperature measurements what enables exact
monitoring of hypothermic patients. Specialised thermometers for core
temperature measurement in oesophagus constitute part of equipment
of all rescue helicopters.

As a part of educational project, National Dispatch staff along with all
members of medical personnel of Polish Medical Air Rescue received educational materials concerning hypothermia and extracorporeal treatment.
Keeping in mind the possibility of further development of hypothermia

treatment program into other areas of Poland, Medical Air Rescue plans to introduce training for medical personnel of all HEMS/EMS centres in Poland on this subject based upon currently introduced e-learning platform.

National Dispatch Office of Polish Medical Air Rescue actively participates in coordination of transportation of patients in severe hypothermia, both from place of incident as well as between medical institutions. Joint experience of Severe Hypothermia Treatment Centre in Kraków and Polish Medical Air Rescue shows that air transport may be the preferable method of translocation of patients in severe hypothermia. Speed, stability and capacity to monitor various aspects of patient's condition are among various advantages of medical helicopter. It is worth noting that despite the slowing of metabolism and prolonged tolerance to hypoxia among hypothermic patients, time of arrival at destination treatment centre remains critical condition for patient's survival chances, like in all other life threatening disorders. It also happens that rescue procedures on site of incident and in emergency ward in hospital takes inadvertently long, so time for transportation is critically shortened. Polish Medical Air Rescue took active part in development of Severe Hypothermia Treatment Centre. Thanks to this, both administration as well as medical personnel may boast good knowledge of protocols of hypothermic patients care, what entails proficiency and high speed at work.

11

Trauma and Hypothermia

Peter Paal[1], Bernd Wallner[2], Hermann Brugger[3]

[1] Head of the Department of Anaesthesiology and Intensive Care Medicine, Hospitallers Brother Hospital, Salzburg, Austria
International Commission for Emergency Medicine (ICAR MEDCOM)
[2] Resident, Department of Anesthesiology and Critical Care Medicine, Innsbruck University Hospital, Austria
PhD Student, Institute of Mountain Emergency Medicine, EURAC Research
[3] Head of the Institute of Mountain Emergency Medicine, EURAC Research
President of the International Society of Mountain Medicine (ISMM)
International Commission for Emergency Medicine (ICAR MEDCOM), Past President

In multiple trauma patients accidental hypothermia (i.e. core temperature < 35°C) is more frequent in winter but must be expected at all seasons of the year, even in regions with moderate climate [1]. The incidence of multiple trauma patients admitted with accidental hypothermia is underestimated, but may exceed 30% [1]. The low reporting rate of accidental hypothermia is partly owed to the lack of reliable thermometers for cold environment. The low awareness for accidental hypothermia leads to insufficient insulation and rewarming measures in the pre- and in-hospital setting.

Accidental hypothermia in multiple trauma is an independent risk factor for increased mortality. In a state-wide trauma registry in Pennsylvania (n = 38,520) mortality of multiple trauma patients increased exponentially with the degree of accidental hypothermia at hospital admission. With a core temperature < 32°C at hospital admission mortality approached 50% (Figure 1) [2]. Multiple trauma patients are prone to accidental hypothermia because central and peripheral thermoregulation are inhibited. This may be due to haemorrhage (i.e. underperfusion of thermoregulation centres in the hypothalamus) and reduced or abolished shivering. Vasodilation as a result of peripheral hypoxia with concomitant metabolic acidosis or analgosedation (possibly less pronounced with ketamine) [3, 4].

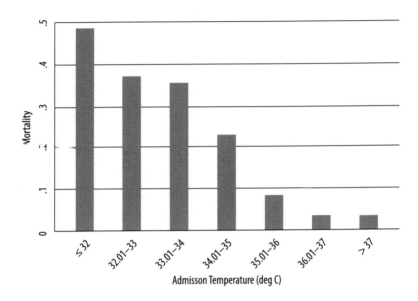

Figure 1. Mortality rates associated with decreasing admission temperatures

Source: Own compilation upon Wang H.E., Callaway C.W., Peitzman A.B., Tisherman S.A. *Admission hypothermia and out-come after major trauma*. Crit. Care Med. 2005; 33: 1296–1301 [2].

Keeping the traumatized patient normothermic is of utmost importance. Patients should be thoroughly and timely insulated, cold and excessive infusions avoided, considerate analgesia and sedation provided with the understanding that they may accelerate cooling. In a cold environment changing clothes is not required as long as patients are insulated water-vapour-tight to avoid heat loss through evaporation [5, 6]. Implementation of the available knowledge and equipment is recommended [7]. Rewarming should be commenced as soon and as aggressively as possible. Even though in regular ambulances and transport times of < 1 hour prehospital rewarming may not be feasible, further cooling of the warm body core by the cold body shell can be limited. In prolonged transports with the availability of forced warm air or heating body pads rewarming (1–2°C/h) may be achieved [8].

A systematic review in elective surgery patients reported that even mild hypothermia (i.e. temperature reduction by 1°C) increased bleeding (+16%) and transfusion requirements (+22%) [9] another study reported similar results in trauma-related laparotomy [10]. Hypothermia, along with acidosis and coagulopathy, is part of the deadly triad in multiple trauma patients and will result in an increase of morbidity and mortality, if not sufficiently counteracted (Figure 2) [11, 12].

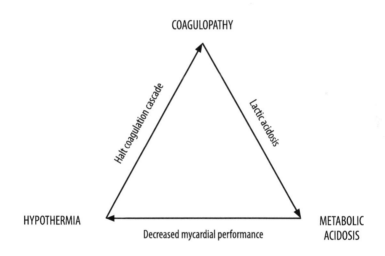

Figure 2. The deadly triad of trauma, consisting of (respiratory and metabolic) acidosis, coagulopathy, and hypothermia

Source: Own elaboration based on *Trauma triad of death*. Wikipedia, 2016 (https://en.wikipedia.org/wiki/Trauma_triad_of_death; accessed: 26.10.2016) [25].

Every decrease in core temperature exponentially increases mortality. Therefore, triaging a multiple trauma patient who is also hypothermic to the right hospital may be lifesaving. Bypassing smaller hospitals on the way to a dedicated trauma centre, ideally equipped with extracorporeal life support, is essential [13]. Immediately after arrival at the hospital aggressive rewarming to normothermia should be initiated to improve circulation and coagulation. Rewarming will ideally start in the trauma department with forced warm air and warm infusions. The operating theatre should be adequately heated to counteract heat loss through extensively uncovered body parts during surgery [8]. Warming mattresses should be provided in the operating theatre and in the intensive care unit to allow for additional continuous rewarming from beneath.

Continuous measurement of the core temperature is a prerequisite for rewarming. This can be performed epitympanically (in awake patients) or oesophageally (in intubated patients) or, increasingly commonly, with an indwelling urinary catheter. Pitfalls in temperature measurement and management (e.g. overwarming) should be avoided with continuous and reliable temperature monitoring, suited devices and trained staff [14].

In patients with primary hypothermic cardiac arrest and multiple trauma, extracorporeal rewarming should be considered [15, 16]. New generation extracorporeal membrane oxygenation (ECMO) systems are fully heparinized and may allow for fast rewarming and circulatory support until return of spontaneous circulation without the risks inherent to systemic heparinization.

If coagulation monitoring is performed at 37°C, as is customary with traditional measurements, coagulopathies related to hypothermia will not be detected. Thus, in hypothermic multiple trauma patients, coagulation analyses should be temperature corrected to the core temperature of a given patient, this can be achieved with ROTEM® or ROTEG® [17].

Positive correlations between hypothermia and increased mortality have been reported in a multitude of patients, e.g. with burns [18], hip fractures [19], ruptured abdominal aortic aneurysm [20], and multiple trauma [21]. Studies also found a positive correlation between the degree of accidental hypothermia, and surgical site infection [22], multi-organ failure [23], and mortality [24].

In conclusion, in a multiple trauma patient pre-hospitally thorough insulation and the prevention of further heat loss is key. Cold infusions should be avoided. In the hospital aggressive active external rewarming and warm infusions to normothermia is crucial. Patients in primary hypothermic cardiac arrest with multiple trauma may be rewarmed with heparinzed ECMO systems while avoiding systemic heparinization.

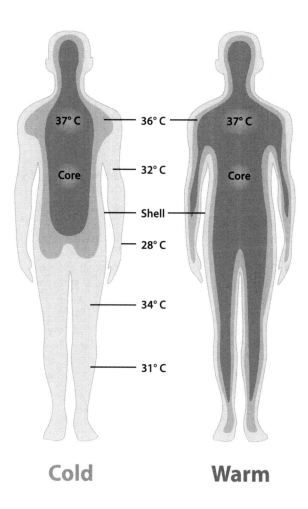

Figure 3. Distribution of temperature in the body between core and periphery during exposure to a cold and a warm environment

Source: Own elaboration based on *Distribution of temperature in the body between core and shelf*. Clinicalgate, 2016 (http://clinicalgate.com/wp-content/uploads/2015/06/B9781437716788000106_f010-001-9781437716788.jpg; accessed: 26.10.2016) [26].

References

1. Mommsen P., Andruszkow H., Fromke C. et al. *Effects of accidental hypothermia on posttraumatic complications and outcome in multiple trauma patients.* Injury 2013; 44: 86–90.
2. Wang H.E., Callaway C.W., Peitzman A.B., Tisherman S.A. *Admission hypothermia and outcome after major trauma.* Crit. Care Med. 2005; 33: 1296–1301.
3. Marland S., Ellerton J., Andolfatto G. et al. *Ketamine: use in anesthesia.* CNS Neurosci. Ther. 2013; 19: 381–389.
4. Soreide K. *Clinical and translational aspects of hypothermia in major trauma patients: from pathophysiology to prevention, prognosis and potential preservation.* Injury 2014; 45: 647–654.
5. Henriksson O., Lundgren P., Kuklane K., Holmer I., Naredi P., Bjornstig U. *Protection against cold in prehospital care: evaporative heat loss reduction by wet clothing removal or the addition of a vapor barrier – a thermal manikin study.* Prehosp. Disaster Med. 2012; 27: 53–58.
6. Henriksson O., Lundgren P.J., Kuklane K. et al. *Protection against cold in prehospital care: wet clothing removal or addition of a vapor barrier.* Wilderness Environ. Med. 2015; 26: 11–20.
7. Paal P., Gordon L., Strapazzon G. et al. *Accidental hypothermia-an update: The content of this review is endorsed by the International Commission for Mountain Emergency Medicine (ICAR MEDCOM).* Scand. J. Trauma Resusc. Emerg. Med. 2016; 24: 111.
8. Brown D.J., Brugger H., Boyd J., Paal P. *Accidental hypothermia.* N. Engl. J. Med. 2012; 367: 1930–1938.
9. Rajagopalan S., Mascha E., Na J., Sessler D.I. *The effects of mild perioperative hypothermia on blood loss and transfusion requirement.* Anesthesiology 2008; 108: 71–77.
10. Bernabei A.F., Levison M.A., Bender J.S. *The effects of hypothermia and injury severity on blood loss during trauma laparotomy.* J. Trauma 1992; 33: 835–839.
11. Martini W.Z. *Coagulopathy by hypothermia and acidosis: mechanisms of thrombin generation and fibrinogen availability.* J. Trauma 2009; 67: 202–208; discussion 8–9.
12. Mikhail J. *The trauma triad of death: hypothermia, acidosis, and coagulopathy.* AACN Clin. Issues 1999; 10: 85–94.
13. Paal P., Brown D.J., Brugger H., Boyd J. *In hypothermic major trauma patients the appropriate hospital for damage control and rewarming may be life saving.* Injury 2013; 44: 1665.
14. Strapazzon G., Procter E., Paal P., Brugger H. *Pre-hospital core temperature measurement in accidental and therapeutic hypothermia.* High Alt. Med. Biol. 2014; 15: 104–111.

15. Darocha T., Kosinski S., Jarosz A., Drwila R. *Extracorporeal Rewarming From Accidental Hypothermia of Patient With Suspected Trauma.* Medicine (Baltimore) 2015; 94: e1086.
16. Sailhamer E.A., Chen Z., Ahuja N. et al. *Profound hypothermic cardiopulmonary bypass facilitates survival without a high complication rate in a swine model of complex vascular, splenic, and colon injuries.* J. Am. Coll. Surg. 2007; 204: 642–653.
17. Douning L.K., Ramsay M.A., Swygert T.H. et al. *Temperature corrected thrombelastography in hypothermic patients.* Anesth. Analg. 1995; 81: 608–611.
18. Hostler D., Weaver M.D., Ziembicki J.A. et al. *Admission temperature and survival in patients admitted to burn centers.* J. Burn Care Res. 2013; 34: 498–506.
19. Faizi M., Farrier A.J., Venkatesan M. et al. *Is body temperature an independent predictor of mortality in hip fracture patients?* Injury 2014; 45: 1942–1945.
20. Janczyk R.J., Howells G.A., Bair H.A., Huang R., Bendick P.J., Zelenock G.B. *Hypothermia is an independent predictor of mortality in ruptured abdominal aortic aneurysms.* Vasc. Endovascular. Surg. 2004; 38: 37–42.
21. Kutcher M.E., Howard B.M., Sperry J.L. et al. *Evolving beyond the vicious triad: Differential mediation of traumatic coagulopathy by injury, shock, and resuscitation.* J. Trauma Acute Care Surg. 2015; 78: 516–523.
22. Seamon M.J., Wobb J., Gaughan J.P., Kulp H., Kamel I., Dempsey D.T. *The effects of intraoperative hypothermia on surgical site infection: an analysis of 524 trauma laparotomies.* Ann. Surg. 2012; 255: 789–795.
23. Beilman G.J., Blondet J.J., Nelson T.R. et al. *Early hypothermia in severely injured trauma patients is a significant risk factor for multiple organ dysfunction syndrome but not mortality.* Ann. Surg. 2009; 249: 845–850.
24. Ireland S., Endacott R., Cameron P., Fitzgerald M., Paul E. *The incidence and significance of accidental hypothermia in major trauma – a prospective observational study.* Resuscitation 2011; 82: 300–306.
25. *Trauma triad of death.* Wikipedia, 2016 (https://en.wikipedia.org/wiki/Trauma_triad_of_death; accessed: 26.10.2016).
26. *Distribution of temperature in the body between core and shelf.* Clinicalgate, 2016 (http://clinicalgate.com/wp-content/uploads/2015/06/B9781437716788000106_f010-001-9781437716788.jpg; accessed: 26.10.2016).

12

Prehospital Management of Avalanche Victims

Hermann Brugger[1], Giacomo Strapazzon[2], Peter Paal[3]

[1] EURAC Institute of Mountain Emergency Medicine, Bozen, Italy; Innsbruck Medical University, Austria; International Commission for Mountain Emergency Medicine ICAR MEDCOM

[2] EURAC Institute of Mountain Emergency Medicine, Bozen, Italy; International Commission for Mountain Emergency Medicine ICAR MEDCOM

[3] Barts Heart Centre, St Bartholomew's Hospital, West Smithfield, Barts Health NHS Trust, Queen Mary University of London, London, United Kingdom; Department of Anaesthesiology and Critical Care Medicine, Innsbruck University Hospital, Innsbruck, Austria; International Commission for Mountain Emergency Medicine ICAR MEDCOM

This chapter is based on following publications:

- Brugger H., Durrer B., Elsensohn F., Paal P., Strapazzon G., Winterberger E., Zafren K., Boyd J. *Resuscitation of avalanche victims: Evidence--based guidelines of the international commission for mountain emergency medicine (ICAR MEDCOM): intended for physicians and other advanced life support personnel.* Resuscitation 2013; 84: 539–546.
- Brugger H., Paal P., Boyd J. *Prehospital resuscitation of the buried avalanche victim.* High Altitude Medicine & Biology 2011; 12: 199–205.
- Truhlář A., Deakin C.D., Soar J., Khalifa G.E., Alfonzo A., Bierens J.J., Brattebo G., Brugger H., Dunning J., Hunyadi-Anticevic S., Koster R.W., Lockey D.J., Lott C., Paal P., Perkins G.D., Sandroni C., Thies K.C., Zideman D.A., Nolan J.P. *European Resuscitation Council Guidelines for Resuscitation 2015: Section 4. Cardiac arrest in special circumstances.* Resuscitation 2015; 95: 148–201.

Summary

In North America and Europe, approximately 165 people die of avalanches per year. Four factors are decisive for survival: grade and duration of burial, presence of a free airway, and severity of trauma. The overall mortality rate is 23%, but 52.4% in completely buried (i.e. head below the snow) victims in contrast to 4.2% in partially buried (i.e. head free) victims. Survival in completely buried victims drops to 30% within the first 35 minutes due to trauma and asphyxia. Thereafter survival decreases more gradually and victims slowly succumb to a trias of hypoxia, hypercapnia and hypothermia if they are able to breath. In the absence of fatal injuries, rescue strategies depend primarily on trauma, duration of burial, the victim's core temperature and the patency of the airway. In 2015, the European Resuscitation Council proposed an algorithm for the management of avalanche victims. With a burial time < 60 minutes (or core temperature ≥ 30°C) rapid extrication and prevention of asphyxia is essential, with adequate airway management and cardiopulmonary resuscitation. With a burial time > 60 minutes or core temperature < 30°C tackling severe hypothermia should be expected. Gentle extrication and continuous core temperature and cardiac monitoring are recommended. Pulseless victims with a patent airway, duration of burial > 60 minutes or a core temperature < 30°C should receive continuous or intermittent cardiopulmonary resuscitation and be transported to a hospital with extracorporeal rewarming facilities.

Introduction

Since 1983, in Europe and North America in average 165 avalanche fatalities have been recorded annually [1], but in developing countries fatalities are presumed to be many times higher. Most avalanche accidents involve skiers, snowboarders, snowshoe walkers [2] and snowmobilers [3]. Most avalanche accidents occur in free, non-secured alpine areas, outside developed ski resorts [4]. The number of persons exposed to avalanche danger is unknown and mortality in the recreational user groups can be only roughly estimated.

Pathophysiology

Mortality

The overall mortality rate of an avalanche accident is 23% [5]; survival depends on the grade of burial (i.e. *partial* if head is free or *complete* if the head is buried under snow), duration of burial, patency of the airway, presence or absence of an air pocket (i.e. any air space in front of mouth and nose with a patent airway) and severity of trauma.

Grade and depth of burial

Avalanche mortality is 52.4% for completely buried victims, and only 4.2% for victims who were not buried or only partially buried; the mean depth of complete burial is approximately one meter [5].

Duration of burial

If a victim is completely buried, survival is inversely related to the duration of burial [5–8]. Survival probability remains higher than 80% up to about 20 minutes post-burial and drops to approximately 30% at 35 minutes. Deaths in the first 20 minutes are mostly attributable to trauma, whereas deaths between 20 and 35 minutes are mainly due to asphyxia, which is the cause of death in approximately 70% of all avalanche fatalities. Longer than 35 minutes, survival is only possible if a victim is not fatally injured and able to breath under the snow [9, 10]. Slowly the victim will succumb to hypoxia, hypercapnia and hypothermia, whereby hypoxia and hypercapnia depend primarily on characteristics of snow [11].

Airway and air pocket

Cases of successful rewarming of severely hypothermic avalanche victims in cardiac arrest without sequelae are rare in literature [12–14]. Most of these victims presented with a clearly visible air space in front of the mouth and nose upon extrication and had a witnessed cardiac arrest. Human and animal experiments demonstrated that during breathing into artificial air pockets in snow, hypoxia and hypercapnia occur with a concomitant respiratory and metabolic acidosis within a few minutes, and the degree of hypoxia depends on the volume of the air pocket, snow density and unidentified individual characteristics [11, 15–17]. The combination of hypoxia, hypercapnia and hypothermia was termed "triple H syndrome" [11].

Cooling rate during burial

A mean core cooling rate of 3.0°C/h has been calculated for the overall time between avalanche burial and hospital admission [12], but the individual cooling rate during snow burial is very variable and ranges from 0.1°C to a maximum of 8.0°C per hour [13]. This implies that hypothermia with a core temperature < 30°C will develop only as early as one hour after avalanche burial [18].

Trauma

Reported mortality from fatal trauma varies in literature. In Austria a trauma mortality of 5.6% has been established [19] (with dislocated cervical spine fractures as the only cause of death), whereas in Canada the rate of trauma as the only cause of death was 24% [20]. Most frequent injuries are found on extremities, chest and spine. Severity of injuries and trauma mortality are highly dependent on the topography of the terrain (e.g., rocky, forested) and snow composition (e.g. heavy, wet) [7].

Causes of death

Autopsy reports confirm that asphyxia remains the most important cause of death [19–22] (~80%), but trauma mortality is increasing (~18%). Hypothermia alone is rarely the sole cause of death (2%) in avalanche victims, but suspected to be underdiagnosed [21, 23]. In most cases hypothermia is associated with asphyxia and trauma.

On-site management

First responders

Search and extrication of the victims should be initiated as early as possible as every minute of burial may be essential for survival. When the head of a victim is free, airway management and combined CPR (chest compressions and ventilation) should be started, if indicated [24, 25]. After extrication the victim should be protected from cold, using all available materials such as aluminum blankets, clothes, bivouac bag, hat and gloves.

Organized rescue

An avalanche accident should prompt a helicopter rescue operation. The risk to the rescue team should be weighed against the expected benefit of the victim. Since the probability of survival decreases over time, it may be justifiable to take greater risk soon after the accident, but less risk after longer burials. The staff should be dressed warmly with complete winter equipment including avalanche safety devices, with a transceiver and ideally an airbag and artificial airway device (AvaLung® or Airsafe®). All medical equipment should be protected from the cold and electronic instruments prepared with full batteries. Rescue bags should include blankets or similar insulation, aluminized wraps, chemical heat packs, thermometers suitable for core temperature reading and cardiac monitoring devices. Standard guidelines have been introduced by the International Commission for Mountain Emergency Medicine ICAR MEDCOM in 2013 [26] and by the European Resuscitation Council (ERC) in 2015 [18]. The ERC-algorithm for the on-site management of avalanche victims is shown in Figure 1.

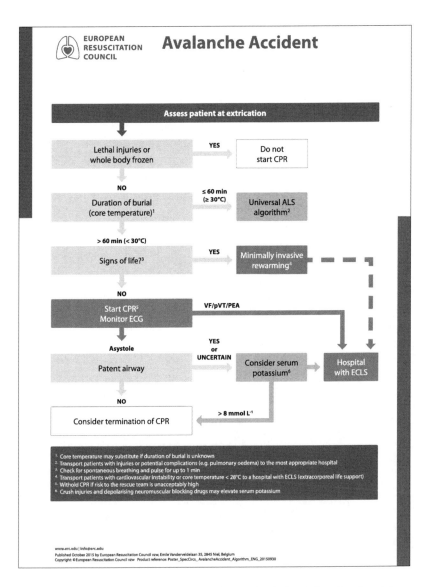

Figure 1. Algorithm for management of completely buried avalanche victims (ECLS – extracorporeal life support)

Source: Own compilation upon Truhlář A., Deakinc C.D., Soar J. et al. *European Resuscitation Council Guidelines for Resuscitation 2015, Section 4. Cardiac arrest in special circumstances*. Resuscitation 2015; 95: 148–201 [18].

Monitoring

A duration of burial of 60 minutes and core temperature of 30°C have been proposed as the thresholds for the initiation of prolonged cardiopulmonary resuscitation (CPR). Early measurement of the core temperature is therefore necessary since the level of consciousness may vary among patients at a given core temperature. The gold standard for core temperature reading is the measurement in the lower third of the oesophagus. If the patient is responsive, epitympanic measurement may be an alternative [27–30]. ECG monitoring should be initiated prior to transport to detect arrhythmias provoked by movement of the patient. Pulse oximetry may be unreliable in hypothermic patients due to peripheral vasoconstriction.

Patient alert and shivering

If the patient is responsive, wet clothing is removed and replaced with dry insulating material and the patient is permitted to walk. Exercise rewarms a person more rapidly than shivering, but may increase afterdrop [17, 31]. Warm drinks may be given providing swallowing is possible. The alert patient without an arrhythmia and with normal blood pressure may be transported to the nearest hospital for observation.

Patient somnolent or comatose but breathing

The three guiding principles for prehospital management of a somnolent or comatose hypothermic patient should be followed: (1) adequate oxygenation, (2) careful handling and (3) full body insulation. Unconscious victims have a low threshold for developing ventricular fibrillation (VF) [32] and require careful handling during rescue and transport. Although it is not always possible to avoid rough movements, movements of the limbs and trunk should be carried out slowly and with great care [33]. Full body insulation and application of hot packs are standard prehospital treatment for hypothermia. Non-intubated patients should receive supplemental oxygen with a facemask or nasal cannula. If the patient is not responsive, the airway should be protected by endotracheal intubation or a supraglottic airway [34, 35]. With low core temperature drug metabolism is decreased and anaesthesia and neuromuscular blockade are prolonged [36–38]. Depolarizing neuromuscular blocking agents (succinylcholine) can affect triage decisions by increasing the serum potassium level (see below). *Victims with severe hypothermia* and circulatory instability (i.e. core temperature < 28°C, ventricular arrhythmias, systolic bloos pressure < 90 mmHg) should be transported to a hospital with extracorporeal life support (ECLS), otherwiese to an intensive care unit experienced in hypothermia care for active external rewarming (e.g. forced air rewarming). In the field, aggressive volume replacement is contraindicated as cardiac output is reduced and the circulating volume contracts due to peripheral vasoconstriction [39]. In patients with a core temperature < 30°C, the administration of advanced life support drugs is controversial and may be withheld [27].

Patient without signs of life

Avalanche victims without vital signs and duration of burial ≤ 60 min or core temperature ≥ 30°C should be treated with Advanced Life Support (ALS). Avalanche victims without vital signs and duration of burial > 60 min or core temperature < 30°C and with a patent airway should be treated as hypothermic patients, managed optimistically and transported in a hospital with ECLS facilities (extracorporeal membrane oxygenation or cardiopulmonary bypass). Detecting vital signs may be difficult in severely hypothermic patients as respiration and pulse may be very slow, irregular and weak. Pulse in hypothermic victims should therefore be checked for up to one minute rather than the 10 seconds recommended for normothermic victims. Any hypothermic avalanche victim with core temperature < 30°C and a patent airway who presents with signs of imminent cardiac arrest (i.e. core temperature < 28°C, ventricular arrhythmia, systolic blood pressure < 90 mmHg) or in cardiac arrest should be transported directly to a centre offering ECLS rewarming [40]. VF may or may not respond to defibrillation < 30°C. Despite this, it may be reasonable to repeat defibrillations, e.g. up to three times [41], but it should be emphasized that if defibrillation attempts are not successful CPR must be continued until extracorporeal rewarming.

CPR

If an avalanche victims presents without vital sings and duration of burial is > 60 min or core temperature < 30°C CPR should be initiated unless the airway is obstructed by snow or debris and the ECG shows asystole. Prolonged CPR should be performed manually or, preferred, using mechanical chest compression devices [18, 42] and the rate of chest compressions and ventilation should be the same as standard basic life support (BLS). If continuous CPR is not possible during transport, delayed or intermittent CPR may be considered (Figure 2) [43]. A patient with cardiac arrest due to primary hypothermia and unknown core temperature or core temperature 20–28°C should receive 5 minutes of CPR alternating with periods of ≤ 5 minutes without CPR. In a patient with core temperature < 20°C, 5 minutes of CPR can be alternated with CPR pauses ≤ 10 minutes.

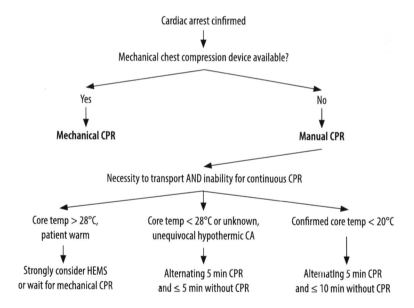

Figure 2. Algorithm for delayed or intermittent CPR in avalanche victims patient with cardiac arrest due to primary hypothermia

Source: Own elaboration based on Gordon L., Paal P., Ellerton J.A., Brugger H., Peek G.J., Zafren K. *Delayed and intermittent CPR for severe accidental hypothermia*. Resuscitation 2015; 90: 46–49 [43].

Serum potassium

Hyperkalaemia is an important outcome marker in avalanche victims [9, 44–51]. For instance, the highest recorded potassium in an avalanche victim who was successfully resuscitated is 6.4 mmol/L [12]. The ERC guidelines 2015 proposed 8.0 mmol/L as threshold for serum potassium [18]. If transport to a unit with ECLS is not readily available, the serum potassium at the nearest hospital en route may be used as prognostic marker whether rewarming should be initiated by any available means.

Avalanche Resuscitation Checklist

A recently published study revealed that adherence to avalanche resuscitation guidelines is poor [52]. In 2015 ICAR MEDCOM proposed the use of an avalanche resuscitation checklist (Figures 3A and 3B) to improve adherence to current guidelines [53]. The checklist has been introduced to improve the outcome of avalanche vitims as well as the data transfer from avalanche to hospital. It should be completed at the site of the accident and should remain with the patient until hospital admission.

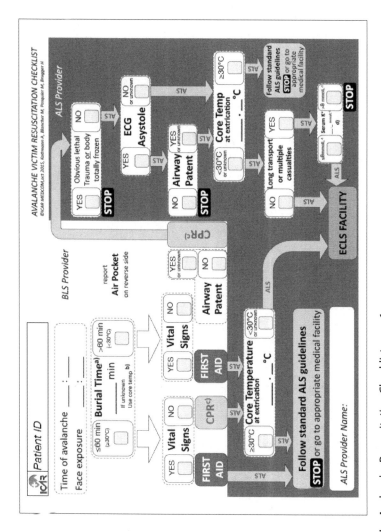

Figure 3A. The Avalanche Resuscitation Checklist page 1

Source: ICAR MEDCOM, OCT. 2015, Kottmann A., Blancher M., Pasquier M., Brugger H.

Air Pocket

☐ Yes, ___ x ___ x ___ (cm)
☐ No
☐ Unknown

Rescue Service:

Base:

Phone:

H The Checklist is to remain with the patient throughout his/her pre-hospital and in-hospital course until final destination.

Rescue Service At Medical Facility delivery, make a copy, a scan or a digital photograph of this checklist and keep it with the copy of your rescue mission protocol.

Abbreviations:
Patient ID = Patient Identity
CPR = Cardiopulmonary Resuscitation
ALS = Advanced Life Support
ECLS = Extra Corporeal Life Support (CardioPulmonary Bypass / Extra Corporeal Membrane Oxygenation)

a) Time between burial and uncovering the face.
b) If duration of burial is unknown, core temperature using an oesophageal probe may substitute in patients in cardiac arrest.
c) CPR can be withheld if unacceptable level of risk for the rescuer, total body frozen or obvious lethal trauma (decapitation, truncal transection).
d) If K^+ at hospital admission exceeds 8 mmolL^{-1} consider terminating resuscitation (after excluding crush injuries and consideration of the use of depolarizing paralytics).

Patients who present with cardiac instability (ventricular arrhythmias, systolic blood pressure <90 mmHg) or core temperature < 30°C should be transported towards hospital with ECLS rewarming possibility.

AVALANCHE VICTIM RESUSCITATION CHECKLIST
ICAR *International Commission for Mountain Emergency medicine*   *www.alpine-rescue.org*
© ICAR, MEDCOM, oct. 2015, Kottmann A, Blancher M, Pasquier M, Brugger H

Figure 3B. The Avalanche Resuscitation Checklist page 2

Source: ICAR MEDCOM, OCT. 2015, Kottmann A., Blancher M., Pasquier M., Brugger H.

Prognosis

The lowest recorded core temperature in an avalanche victim who survived was 19°C [14]. Three retrospective observational studies have found survival rates of avalanche victims who received prolonged CPR ECLS to be 0% (n = 8) [54], 7.1% (n = 28) [47] and 16.7% (n = 48) [55], overall 11%. Survival from cardiac arrest with avalanche burial is lower when compared to hypothermia from other causes, for example environmental exposure including cold water immersion [40, 56, 57]. This is very likely related to the faster cooling rates in persons exposed to the latter conditions compared to commonly well insulated people buried by avalanches.

Termination of CPR

If an avalanche victims presents with cardiac arrest and duration of burial is ≤ 60 min, resuscitation may be terminated if ALS is not successful after limited time. Resuscitation is also not indicated if the victim presents with a lethal injury, with an obstructed airway and asystole after more than one hour burial, if chest is incompressible, or if CPR would endanger the rescuers [58]. In all other cases the guiding principle should be "no hypothermic avalanche victim with a patent airway is dead until warm and dead" [23].

Disclosure

No financial conflict of interest.

References

1. International Commission for Alpine Rescue ICAR. *Avalanche deaths by country and activity sind 1983 in Europe and North America* (http://wwwalpine-rescueorg/xCMS5/WebObjects/nexus5woa/wa/icar?menuid=1067&rubricid=263&articleid=12597; accessed: 5.07.2016).

2. Procter E., Strapazzon G., Dal Cappello T., Castlunger L., Staffler H.P., Brugger H. *Adherence of backcountry winter recreationists to avalanche prevention and safety practices in northern Italy.* Scand. J. Med. Sci. Sports. 2014; 24: 823–829.
3. Stethem C., Jamieson B., Schaerer P., Liverman D., Germain D., Walker S. *Snow avalanche hazard in Canada – A review.* Nat. Hazards 2003; 28: 487–515.
4. Hohlrieder M., Thaler S., Wuertl W., Voelckel W., Ulmer H., Brugger H., Mair P. *Rescue missions for totally buried avalanche victims: conclusions from 12 years of experience.* High Alt. Med. Biol. 2008; 9: 229–233.
5. Brugger H., Durrer B., Adler-Kastner L., Falk M., Tschirky F. *Field management of avalanche victims.* Resuscitation 2001; 51: 7–15.
6. Falk M., Brugger H., Adler-Kastner L. *Avalanche survival chances.* Nature 1994; 368: 21.
7. Haegeli P., Falk M., Brugger H., Etter H.J., Boyd J. *Comparison of avalanche survival patterns in Canada and Switzerland.* CMAJ 2011; 183: 789–795.
8. Procter E., Strapazzon G., Dal Cappello T., Zweifel B., Wurtele A. Renner A., Falk M., Brugger H. *Burial duration, depth and air pocket explain avalanche survival patterns in Austria and Switzerland.* Resuscitation 2016; 105: 173–176.
9. Boyd J., Brugger H., Shuster M. *Prognostic factors in avalanche resuscitation: a systematic review.* Resuscitation 2010; 81: 645–652.
10. Soar J., Perkins G.D., Abbas G., Alfonzo A., Barelli A., Bierens J.J., Brugger H., Deakin C.D., Dunning J., Georgiou M., Handley A.J., Lockey D.J., Paal P., Sandroni C., Thies K.C., Zideman D.A., Nolan J.P. *European Resuscitation Council Guidelines for Resuscitation 2010 Section 8. Cardiac arrest in special circumstances: Electrolyte abnormalities, poisoning, drowning, accidental hypothermia, hyperthermia, asthma, anaphylaxis, cardiac surgery, trauma, pregnancy, electrocution.* Resuscitation 2010; 81: 1400–1433.
11. Brugger H., Sumann G., Meister R., Adler-Kastner L., Mair P., Gunga H.C., Schobersberger W., Falk M. *Hypoxia and hypercapnia during respiration into an artificial air pocket in snow: implications for avalanche survival.* Resuscitation 2003; 58: 81–88.
12. Locher T., Walpoth B.H. *Differential diagnosis of circulatory failure in hypothermic avalanche victims: retrospective analysis of 32 avalanche accidents.* Praxis (Bern 1994) 1996; 85: 1275–1282.
13. Oberhammer R., Beikircher W., Hormann C., Lorenz I., Pycha R., Adler-Kastner L., Brugger H. *Full recovery of an avalanche victim with profound hypothermia and prolonged cardiac arrest treated by extracorporeal re-warming.* Resuscitation 2008; 76: 474–480.
14. Althaus U., Aeberhard P., Schupbach P., Nachbur B.H., Muhlemann W. *Management of profound accidental hypothermia with cardiorespiratory arrest.* Annals of Surgery 1982; 195: 492–495.

15. Grissom C.K., Radwin M.I., Harmston C.H. *Improving survival during snow burial in avalanches.* JAMA 2000; 284: 1242–1243.
16. Grissom C.K., Radwin M.I., Scholand M.B., Harmston C.H., Muetterties M.C., Bywater T.J. *Hypercapnia increases core temperature cooling rate during snow burial.* J. Appl. Phys. 2004; 96: 1365–1370.
17. Grissom C.K., McAlpine J.C., Harmston C.H., Radwin M.I., Giesbrecht G.G., Scholand M.B., Morgan J.S. *Hypercapnia effect on core cooling and shivering threshold during snow burial.* Aviat. Space Environ. Med. 2008; 79: 735–742.
18. Truhlář A., Deakin C.D., Soar J., Khalifa G.E.A., Alfonzo A., Bierens J., Brattebøh G., Brugger H., Dunningj J., Hunyadi-Antičević S., Koster R.W., Lockey D.J., Lottn C., Paal P., Perkins G.D., Sandroni C., Thiest K.C., Zideman D.A., Nolan J.P. *European Resuscitation Council Guidelines for Resuscitation 2015 Section 4. Cardiac arrest in special circumstances.* Resuscitation 2015; 95: 148–201.
19. Hohlrieder M., Brugger H., Schubert H.M., Pavlic M., Ellerton J., Mair P. *Pattern and severity of injury in avalanche victims.* High Alt. Med. Biol. 2007; 8: 56–61.
20. Boyd J., Haegeli P., Abu-Laban R.B., Shuster M., Butt J.C. *Patterns of death among avalanche fatalities: a 21-year review.* CMAJ 2009; 180: 507–512.
21. Brugger H., Etter H.J., Boyd J., Falk M. *Causes of death from avalanche.* Wilderness Environ. Med. 2009; 20: 93–96.
22. McIntosh S.E., Grissom C.K., Olivares C.R., Kim H.S., Tremper B. *Cause of death in avalanche fatalities.* Wilderness Environ. Med. 2007; 18: 293–297.
23. Brugger H., Paal P., Boyd J. *Prehospital resuscitation of the buried avalanche victim.* High Alt. Med. Biol. 2011; 12: 199–205.
24. Nolan J.P., Soar J., Zideman D.A., Biarent D., Bossaert L.L., Deakin C., Koster R.W., Wyllie J., Böttiger B. *European Resuscitation Council Guidelines for Resuscitation 2010 Section 1. Executive summary.* Resuscitation 2010; 81: 1219–1276.
25. Berg R.A., Hemphill R., Abella B.S., Aufderheide T.P., Cave D.M., Hazinski M.F., Lerner E.B., Rea T.D., Sayre M.R., Swor R.A. *Part 5: adult basic life support: 2010 American Heart Association Guidelines for Cardiopulmonary Resuscitation and Emergency Cardiovascular Care.* Circulation 2010; 122: S685–S705.
26. Brugger H., Durrer B., Elsensohn F., Paal P., Strapazzon G., Winterberger E., Zafren K., Boyd J. *Resuscitation of avalanche victims: Evidence-based guidelines of the international commission for mountain emergency medicine (ICAR MEDCOM): intended for physicians and other advanced life support personnel.* Resuscitation 2013; 84: 539–546.
27. Walpoth B.H., Galdikas J., Leupi F., Muehlemann W., Schlaepfer P., Althaus U. *Assessment of hypothermia with a new "tympanic" thermometer.* J. Clin. Monit. 1994; 10: 91–96.
28. Strapazzon G., Procter E., Paal P., Brugger H. *Pre-hospital core temperature measurement in accidental and therapeutic hypothermia.* High Alt. Med. Biol. 2014; 15: 104–111.

29. Strapazzon G., Procter E., Putzer G., Avancini G., Dal Cappello T., Uberbacher N., Hofer G., Rainer B., Rammlmair G., Brugger H. *Influence of low ambient temperature on epitympanic temperature measurement: a prospective randomized clinical study.* Scand. J. Trauma Resusc. Emerg. Med. 2015; 23: 90.

30. Strapazzon G., Procter E., Avancini G., Überbacher N., Putzer G., Hofer G., Rainer B., Dal Cappello T., Ledoux X., Brugger H. *Thermistor probe for measurement of tympanic temperature: Influence of ambient temperature.* Resuscitation 2013; 84S: S93.

31. Giesbrecht G.G., Bristow G.K. *Recent advances in hypothermia research.* Annals of the New York Academy of Sciences 1997; 813: 663–675.

32. Danzl D.F., Pozos R.S. *Accidental hypothermia.* N. Engl. J. Med. 1994; 331: 1756–1760.

33. Kornberger E., Mair P. *Important aspects in the treatment of severe accidental hypothermia: the Innsbruck experience.* J. Neurosurg. Anesthesiol. 1996; 8: 83–87.

34. Deakin C.D., Nolan J.P., Soar J., Sunde K., Koster R.W., Smith G.B., Perkins G.D. *European Resuscitation Council Guidelines for Resuscitation 2010 Section 4. Adult advanced life support.* Resuscitation 2010; 81: 1305–1352.

35. Morrison L.J., Deakin C.D., Morley P.T., Callaway C.W., Kerber R.E., Kronick S.L., Lavonas E.J., Link M.S., Neumar R.W., Otto C.W., Parr M., Shuster M., Sunde K., Peberdy M.A., Tang W., Hoek T.L., Bottiger B.W., Drajer S., Lim S.H., Nolan J.P. *Part 8: Advanced life support: 2010 International Consensus on Cardiopulmonary Resuscitation and Emergency Cardiovascular Care Science With Treatment Recommendations.* Circulation 2010; 122: S345–S421.

36. Leslie K., Sessler D.I., Bjorksten A.R., Moayeri A. *Mild hypothermia alters Propofol pharmacokinetics and increases the duration of action of Atracurium.* Anesth. Analg. 1995; 80: 1007–1014.

37. Caldwell J.E., Heier T., Wright P.M., Lin S., McCarthy G., Szenohradszky J., Sharma M.L., Hing J.P., Schroeder M., Sessler D.I. *Temperature-dependent pharmacokinetics and pharmacodynamics of vecuronium.* Anesthesiology 2000; 92: 84–93.

38. Heier T., Caldwell J.E. *Impact of hypothermia on the response to neuromuscular blocking drugs.* Anesthesiology 2006; 104: 1070–1080.

39. Lloyd E.L. *The cause of death after rescue.* Int. J. Sports Med. 1992; 13: 196–199.

40. Brown D.J., Brugger H., Boyd J., Paal P. *Accidental hypothermia.* N. Engl. J. Med. 2012; 367: 1930–1938.

41. Vanden Hoek T.L., Morrison L.J., Shuster M., Donnino M., Sinz E., Lavonas E.J., Jeejeebhoy F.M., Gabrielli A. *Part 12: cardiac arrest in special situations: 2010 American Heart Association Guidelines for Cardiopulmonary Resuscitation and Emergency Cardiovascular Care.* Circulation 2010; 122: S829–S861.

42. Putzer G., Braun P., Zimmermann A., Pedross F., Strapazzon G., Brugger H., Paal P. *LUCAS compared to manual cardiopulmonary resuscitation is more effective during helicopter rescue-a prospective, randomized, cross-over manikin study.* Am. J. Emerg. Med. 2012; 31: 384–389.

43. Gordon L., Paal P., Ellerton J.A., Brugger H., Peek G.J., Zafren K. *Delayed and intermittent CPR for severe accidental hypothermia.* Resuscitation 2015; 90: 46–49.
44. Schaller M.D., Fischer A.P., Perret C.H. *Hyperkalemia. A prognostic factor during acute severe hypothermia.* JAMA 1990; 264: 1842–1845.
45. Locher T., Walpoth B., Pfluger D., Althaus U. *Accidental hypothermia in Switzerland (1980–1987) – case reports and prognostic factors.* Schweiz Med. Wochenschr. 1991; 121: 1020–1028.
46. Mair P., Kornberger E., Furtwaengler W., Balogh D., Antretter H. *Prognostic markers in patients with severe accidental hypothermia and cardiocirculatory arrest.* Resuscitation 1994; 27: 47–54.
47. Mair P., Brugger H., Mair B., Moroder L., Ruttmann E. *Is extracorporeal rewarming indicated in avalanche victims with unwitnessed hypothermic cardiorespiratory arrest?* High Alt. Med. Biol. 2014; 15: 500–503.
48. Blancher M., Boussat B., Bouzat P. *Blood potassium after avalanche-induced cardiac arrest: sampling method and interpretation.* Am. J. Emerg. Med. 2016; 34: 1317–1318.
49. Briot R., Blancher M. *Accidental Hypothermia Cardiac Arrest. Keeping High Hyperkalemia Cut-Off?* Crit. Care Med. 2016; 44: e593.
50. Cohen J.G., Boue Y., Boussat B., Reymond E., Grand S., Blancher M., Ferretti G.R., Bouzat P. *Serum potassium concentration predicts brain hypoxia on CT after avalanche-induced cardiac arrest.* Am. J. Emerg. Med. 2016; 34: 856–860.
51. Strapazzon G., Falk M., Paal P., Brugger H. *The challenge of establishing a correct serum potassium cutoff for inhospital triage after avalanche-induced cardiac arrest.* Am. J. Emerg. Med. 2016; 34: 1317.
52. Strapazzon G., Plankensteiner J., Mair P., Ruttmann E., Brugger H. *Triage and survival of avalanche victims with out-of-hospital cardiac arrest in Austria between 1987 and 2009.* Resuscitation 2012; 83: e81.
53. Kottmann A., Blancher M., Spichiger T., Elsensohn F., Letang D., Boyd J., Strapazzon G., Ellerton J., Brugger H. *The Avalanche Victim Resuscitation Checklist, a new concept for the management of avalanche victims.* Resuscitation 2015; 9: e7–e8.
54. Hilmo J., Naesheim T., Gilbert M. *"Nobody is dead until warm and dead": Prolonged resuscitation is warranted in arrested hypothermic victims also in remote areas – A retrospective study from northern Norway.* Resuscitation 2014; 85: 1204–1211.
55. Boue Y., Payen J.F., Brun J., Thomas S., Levrat A., Blancher M., Debaty G., Bouzat P. *Survival after avalanche-induced cardiac arrest.* Resuscitation 2014; 85: 1192–1196.
56. Walpoth B.H., Walpoth-Aslan B.N., Mattle H.P., Radanov B.P., Schroth G., Schaeffler L., Fischer A.P., von Segesser L., Althaus U. *Outcome of survivors of accidental deep hypothermia and circulatory arrest treated with extracorporeal blood warming.* N. Engl. J. Med. 1997; 337: 1500–1505.

57. Wanscher M., Agersnap L., Ravn J., Yndgaard S., Nielsen J.F., Danielsen E.R., Hassager C., Romner B., Thomsen C., Barnung S., Lorentzen A.G., Hogenhaven H., Davis M., Moller J.E. *Outcome of accidental hypothermia with or without circulatory arrest: experience from the Danish Praesto Fjord boating accident.* Resuscitation 2012; 83: 1078–1084.

58. Paal P., Milani M., Brown D., Boyd J., Ellerton J. *Termination of cardiopulmonary resuscitation in mountain rescue.* High Alt. Med. Biol. 2012; 13: 200–208.

13

Prehospital Rewarming in Hypothermia. Indications, Methods, Problems and Pitfalls

Les Gordon

Consultant Anaesthetist, University Hospitals of Morecambe Bay Trust, Lancaster, England
Team Doctor, Langdale Ambleside Mountain Rescue Team, England

Introduction

Understanding the clinical classification of hypothermia helps with all aspects of management, of which rewarming is a part. The original Swiss classification published in 2003 [1] has been updated [2].

Table 1. Update Swiss Staging System

Stage	Clinical Findings	Core temperature (if available)
Hypothermia I (mild) HT I	conscious; shivering	35–32°C
Hypothermia II (moderate) HT II	impaired consciousness; may or may not be shivering	< 32–28°C
Hypothermia III (severe) HT III	unconscious; vital signs present	< 28°C
Hypothermia IV (severe) HT IV	apparent death; vital signs absent	Variable

Source: Own compiled upon Brown D.J.A. *Hypothermia*. In: Tintinalli J.E. ed. *Emergency Medicine*. 8th ed. McGraw Hill, New York 2015: 1357–1365 [2].

Important notes [3]

- Shivering and consciousness (HT I–III) may be impaired by comorbid illness (i.e. trauma, medical conditions, etc.) or drugs (i.e. sedatives, narcotics, alcohol, etc.) independent of core temperature. The lowest temperature from which successful resuscitation and rewarming has been achieved is currently 13.7°C [4] for accidental hypothermia and 9°C [5] for induced hypothermia. This does not preclude resuscitation attempts at even lower temperatures if clinical judgement suggests the possibility of successful resuscitation.
- The risk of cardiac arrest (HT IV) increases below 32°C. However, it is unlikely to be due solely to hypothermia until the temperature is < 28°C so alternative causes should be considered. Some patients still have vital signs well below 24°C. The lowest reported temperature of a patient with vital signs is 17°C.

Although rewarming all hypothermic victims is essential, how this is done, by how much and how effective it will be in the prehospital environment depends primarily on the stage of hypothermia, but also on any associated medical conditions the patient has, the rescuer's level of training, the resuscitation equipment available, type of transportation, and time required for delivery to definitive care. In all cases, the first steps are to stop/minimise further heat loss by providing shelter, removing wet clothes (when appropriate), insulation from the ground and protection from wind (including helicopter downwash) and rain. After that, in HT I, full care can proceed (discussed below). However, large physiological changes will usually have occurred by the time core temperature has fallen to < 28°C, so in these patients, although there are no restrictions on the amount of insulation that may be used, other options are more limited. A vapour barrier should be used to contain endogenous heat, and exogenous heat application should only be sufficient to arrest the cooling process or provide minimal rewarming to prevent a further fall in cardiac temperature. Full rewarming should take place in the controlled environment of a hospital when the issues of body temperature, hydration, substrate depletion, arrhythmia management, respiratory compromise, frostbite, plus any other problems e.g. comorbid illness, drug/alcohol ingestion, trauma will be simultaneously addressed.

Mild hypothermia

Although the magnitude and effectiveness of the overall physiological response to cold depends on many patient factors (e.g. age, body habitus, concurrent disease, trauma, intoxication, analgesia, sedation, etc.) [6], in mild hypothermia (HT I; 35–32°C), shivering combined with active movement are very efficient mechanisms of heat production and are good rewarming strategies for patients who are fully conscious and able to move [7–9]. Exercise can achieve a rate of core-temperature rise (°C per hour) that is ≈40% greater than the application of external heat or shivering [9]. External heat is slightly more effective than shivering [9]. At rest, shivering can increase heat production by up to 5 times the resting metabolic rate [10] leading to a temperature rise of 3–4°C/h [11]. Although this is at the expense of increased oxygen requirements [8, 12], it is unlikely to be a problem in an uninjured person with normal cardiorespiratory function. Due to the body's ability to use a wide range of energy substrates [8, 13], a high level of shivering heat production can be maintained for ≈4–6 hours before it starts to decline [14]. This will occur when the core--temperature drops below an individual's threshold, which is generally ≈30°C [15] (although this depends on many factors [8] including fatigue [16]) or when energy stores are depleted [6, 8]. A warm, sweet, non-alcoholic drink will not provide enough heat to rewarm a HT I patient but will supply some carbohydrate to fuel continued shivering [17–19].

In addition to shivering, insulation from the environment, exchanging wet clothes for dry and the application of heat are all extremely beneficial [7]. Exogenous skin heating is equally effective whether applied to the head or torso [20]. It makes the patient feel better but reduces shivering heat production [9] by an amount equivalent to the heat applied [21–23]. It therefore may not rewarm more quickly than shivering [9, 11, 23, 24]. The reduction of shivering by exogenous heat does have the advantages of reducing cardiac work and preserving energy substrate reserves [22]. In the absence of exogenous heat, experimental evidence suggests that mildly hypothermic victims who are otherwise healthy and shivering vigorously can be provided with general support (dry clothes, insulation, protection from the elements and food) and allowed to continue to shiver [9, 21]. This does not apply to victims who have stopped shivering, when exogenous heat would be beneficial [9]. It is not possible to rewarm the whole body by inhaling warmed air due to inability to safely deliver sufficient heat [25–28], but it will produce localised tissue rewarming [29] and will reduce respiratory heat losses [11, 17, 27].

Afterdrop

Afterdrop is a continued fall in core temperature despite removal from the cold stress and application of insulation [30]. It should be distinguished from the continued cooling, that occurs when victims have been removed from a cold environment (e.g. water) but inadequately insulated, with further cooling occurring e.g. due to the wind [30]. Afterdrop has been well documented and researched for many years [11, 23, 31]. It is seen after rescue, during transport [28], during rewarming in the prehospital and hospital environments [9, 32, 33] and also during rewarming from hypothermia for cardiac surgery [34–36].

The precise mechanism by which afterdrop occurs is unclear. It used to be thought that the application of external heat to a moderate-severely hypothermic patient would be hazardous because it would cause sudden peripheral vasodilation and allow cold blood to return to the core, thereby causing a fall in core temperature (afterdrop) and precipitating VF [28]. However, there is no evidence to support this theory [11, 28], perhaps because perfusion of the extremities is not re-established during rewarming until the deep body temperature is > 35°C [37]. Even placing the arms and legs of a hypothermic patient in water at 45°C does not lead to a fall in core temperature [38].

There appear to be two processes underlying the phenomenon. Heat loss continues from deeper tissues to the periphery by conduction [31, 32, 39]. Therefore, afterdrop detection and magnitude will depend on where the temperature is measured [29, 30]. It will be more pronounced at sites that are primarily dependent on conductive heat exchange, such as the nasopharynx and rectum, than at sites where temperature is primarily determined by flow, such as the heart [30]. Even so, afterdrop has been documented in the heart [29]. Secondly, blood flow to cooler tissue in the peripheries subsequently returns to and cools the central circulation and the heart [29, 32, 40]. This is enhanced by exercise-assisted rewarming due to increased blood flow through cold muscle [9, 40, 41], and also by passive limb movements (e.g. raising the legs) or rubbing the arms and legs, a change in posture (so the casualty should be kept horizontal [11]) or the cessation of "hydrostatic pressure" when a casualty is removed from water [28]. This "convective" mechanism will result in greater cooling than by conduction [32], unless the patient is in cardiac arrest (CA).

The reported magnitude of afterdrop depends on several factors but can be as much as 5–6°C [11, 32]. It is therefore potentially clinically relevant in victims who are at the threshold of moderate to severe hypothermia because cardiac instability could occur with just a small fall in core temperature. Experimental studies have demonstrated a small afterdrop (£1°C) during minimally-invasive rewarming [23, 29, 40, 41]. Shivering [42] and the application of exogenous heat attenuate the amount and duration of afterdrop [23, 43]. Interestingly, case reports suggest that afterdrop is less likely to occur if body rewarming is slow (£2°C/h) [44–52], which makes sense as the whole body warms as a single unit rather than with some areas well ahead of others [29, 39]. Afterdrop may be more likely with rapid rewarming [29] e.g. ≈5°C/h with exercise [9] and this has led some experts to argue that hypothermic patients should neither stand nor walk for 30 minutes after rescue-care commences [7]. This could be particularly important when hypothermia is more severe (< 32°C), if core temperature is unknown, and in people who are physically and/or metabolically exhausted and therefore incapable of shivering. In these individuals, a slower less stressful form of rewarming must be used [9]. In mild hypothermia, patients rewarm faster in the exercise group because of a greater capacity to generate heat (as discussed above) and as no adverse outcomes have ever been observed in either group, patients who are awake and alert should not be prevented from mobilising if this will help the rescue [53, 54].

Moderate and severe hypothermia (core temperature < 32°C)

The issues of stopping further heat loss and rewarming become much more critical when core temperature is < 32°C and the victim has stopped shivering. When shivering ceases (HT II–IV), minimal rewarming occurs [42] and in the absence of adequate insulation and heat during transport, cooling will continue [23, 26, 28], thereby increasing the risk of CA. Therefore, the primary goals of the prehospital management of victims with severe hypothermia are the prevention of CA e.g. by careful handling, and the prevention or limiting of a further fall in core temperature as this will increase the likelihood of CA.

Important physiological issues in severe hypothermia and implications for rewarming in the prehospital situation

Many physiological changes occur in hypothermia and these are well described elsewhere [17, 28]. A few are particularly relevant in relation to prehospital rewarming:

- Animal experiments have shown that myocardial cooling from 30°C to 22°C causes a five-fold decrease in the electrical threshold for VF [55, 56]. Therefore, a priority is to at least attempt to stop further cardiac cooling, if not reverse it.
- Peripheral vasoconstriction initially results in central hypervolaemia, leading to a diuresis and intravascular dehydration [17, 28]. Therefore warmed intravenous fluids [17, 57], potentially in large volumes, will be needed to accommodate the increasing size of the vascular bed as the patient rewarms [71]. There is animal evidence that replacement of fluids before rewarming augments cardiac output [58]. It is therefore essential not to attempt significant rewarming in the absence of adequate fluid replacement.
- The vasoconstriction is so intense that only massive heating by immersion in warm water will overcome it, which is why the vasodilation theory mentioned above has been discounted. Therefore, any heat source that can function in the prehospital situation is probably safe [11]. In particular, it is now recognised that gradual core rewarming through the application of heat to the chest and axillae is valuable as long as cardiovascular stability is maintained [11].
- Respiratory function deteriorates as body temperature falls. This includes a fall in minute volume and ventilation-perfusion mismatch [17]. Although oxygen consumption falls with hypothermia, it will in-

crease with rise in temperature. Therefore adequate oxygen supplementation is essential during rewarming.

- Hypothermia protects the brain so ideally, it should not be rewarmed until the circulation is stable enough to maintain an effective continuous cerebral blood flow. Some experts even recommend shielding the head from external heat sources to prevent the brain temperature from rising too quickly until the circulation has stabilised [3]. The greatest danger would be partial rewarming e.g. from a core temperature 22°C to 28°C, followed by a prehospital CA, perhaps triggered by patient movement.

Practical considerations

Evidence-based guidelines for prehospital rewarming do not exist but many human studies have compared insulation and/or heating methods [9, 19, 21–24, 49, 59–62, 66, 68–70]. A multi-layered metalized plastic sheeting survival bag may be beneficial in less severe cases of hypothermia, particularly if combined with heat pads [19]. However, in more severe cases, experimental evidence and experience indicate that pre-hospital patient packaging should include a sealed impermeable vapour barrier [61] for prevention of convective and evaporative heat loss [28, 59] (especially if the patient is wet) covering the whole body but excluding the face [63], an external heat source, dry insulation (the thicker, the better), and a wind barrier that also reflects heat [59]. These are discussed further below.

Insulation

Efforts should be made to minimise all sources of heat loss by maximum insulation from the cold, wet, and wind as soon as possible [11]. It is important that the outer layer is windproof and compression resistant to maintain adequate insulation capacity, particularly in prolonged rescues [62]. Insulation is also particularly important when removing an avalanche victim, as the cooling rate after extrication is faster than during burial [64].

Removal of wet clothing

Manikin and human experiments have confirmed that wet clothing con-
ducts heat away from the body much faster than dry, so it is preferable to remove it when possible and replace it with dry clothing [60, 62].
If the body temperature is < 32°C, it is important to balance the risks of
removing the clothing (increased cooling during removal or triggering an
arrhythmia if the body is handled roughly) against leaving wet clothing
in place. If the decision is taken to remove the clothing, this must only
be done if adequate shelter can be provided, as otherwise, it will result in
rapid cooling if done in a cold/windy environment [1, 60, 61]. Carefully cut
off the clothes, removing a bit at a time rather than all at once, to minimise
further cooling and patient movement [11]. If possible, the patient's skin
should be dried using gentle blotting motions (not by rubbing, as this can
increase circulation to cold limbs as described above) and then dry insulating clothing put on, followed by a layer of insulation (blankets, sleeping
bag, etc.) and finally, an outer impermeable vapour barrier (see below)
that will protect the insulation from becoming wet [11].

Vapour barrier

A vapour barrier is an occlusive sheet covering the insulation and it can
substantially reduce heat loss in adverse conditions. It is of particular value in a cold environment, in the presence of wet clothes [59, 60, 62] or
when limited insulation is available. It should be sealed but allow access
where necessary. There are occasions when clothing removal will be ri-
sky e.g. due to physical location, because of patient injuries (e.g. spinal) or
when temperature is < 32°C, as described above. Although removing wet
clothes increases patient comfort, it is thermally unnecessary if a vapour
barrier is used [60, 62]. If it is deemed safer to leave wet clothes in place
until the casualty is in a warm environment (e.g. vehicle or (better) hospital), the vapour barrier should be applied around the patient and inside
the layers of insulation [11].
    The vapour barrier has two functions. It is a physical barrier to the we-
ather. Secondly, it minimises heat loss. Once the atmosphere inside the
enclosure is fully saturated with water vapour, no more heat can be lost by

evaporation from the skin or by convection, which are the major routes of heat loss in this situation [59, 65].

Reflective blankets have little additional value over a heavy-duty plastic bag as little heat loss occurs by radiation because the skin temperature is so low [65–67]. Furthermore, the ability to radiate heat back to the body by a reflective surface may be compromised by evaporated (possibly exhaled) water condensing on the inner layer of the bag, causing the reflective properties to be lost [65].

Bubble wrap has been used by some emergency services. It is light-weight and water-resistant, but is available in different thicknesses with different insulation properties so it is hard to give a description that covers all. However, research evidence suggests that in spite of its popularity, it is actually of limited use on its own [59, 62, 68–70].

Heat sources

In severe hypothermia when shivering has ceased, little or no rewarming will occur without the application of external heat [23]. Applying heat increases patient comfort [22]. Medical indications for applying heat include [17]:

* cardiovascular instability;
* moderate/severe hypothermia (< 32°C; HT II–IV);
* inadequate rate or failure to rewarm spontaneously;
* accompanying medical, trauma or toxicological problems.

Body-to-body rewarming is neither practical nor very effective and is not generally recommended [11]. Heat-generating devices are very useful in austere environments. They will help to stabilise and even raise slightly the core temperature in patients who have stopped shivering [11]. It is appropriate to apply heat from the incident site and during transport, particularly if the journey will take > 30 minutes [11]. Heat should be applied to the head [20] (if the circulation is stable – see above), thorax and neck areas [11, 23, 28, 71], as the skin blood flow in these areas is less affected by temperature, unlike the limbs [23]. Heat must never be applied directly to skin because of the risk of burns [28]. This occurs because circulation in the skin is so poor that even a low level of heat is not conducted away, but builds up. Patients in CA (HT IV) being transported for ECLS-rewarming should ideally have their core-temperature monitored and heat delivery should be titrated to maintain the core body temperature. Prehospital rewarming or cooling of HT IV during transport should be avoided [3] if possible.

There is a range of heating options for the prehospital situation. Importantly, the first two start off hot but cool and may need replenishing during a prolonged evacuation:

- chemical heat-packs [19, 22, 23, 68, 72];
- warm water bottles [23];
- charcoal heater [23, 43];
- forced air blankets [11, 17, 26, 43, 46] are very effective; small units are available that can work in a prehospital setting such as an aircraft but require a mains power supply [73].

A low-tech variant on the above is Hibler's method [74]. The Principle involves soaking a towel in water at 40°C and placing it on the victim's chest, then covering with a plastic sheet (vapour barrier) and insulation. But even insulation and vapour barrier alone are effective [59, 75].

Warmed intravenous fluids (≈40°C) can be given to help maintain the circulation [28]. This will not provide enough heat to significantly rewarm the victim [76], but at least will not exacerbate cooling. It has been calculated that at 40°C, 10 litres of fluid would be required to increase the body temperature by 1°C [77] – something that is not achievable in the prehospital situation.

Severe hypothermia in the patient with cardiac arrest

If a mechanical chest compression device is available, do not place the patient on it until CA occurs, thereby reducing the pressure on the patient's skin from the hard board and making the stretcher lighter. However, packaging should be flexible enough to allow the patient to be transported on the device with it in use.

Conclusion

Understanding the issues should enable practitioners to deliver optimal rewarming in the prehospital situation, particularly in severe hypothermia. The most important factors are protection from the environment, maximum insulation, restoring body energy stores when possible, prevention of CA e.g. by careful handling, and the prevention or limiting of a further fall in core temperature as this will increase the likelihood of CA.

References

1. Durrer B., Brugger H., Syme D. *The medical on-site treatment of hypothermia: ICAR-MEDCOM recommendation.* High Alt. Med. Biol. 2003; 4: 99–103.
2. Brown D.J.A. *Hypothermia.* In: Tintinalli J.E. ed. *Emergency Medicine.* 8th ed. McGraw Hill, New York 2015: 1357–1365.
3. Paal P., Gordon L., Strapazzon G., Maeder M.B., Putzer G., Walpoth B., Wanscher M., Brown D., Holzer M., Broessner G., Brugger H. *Accidental hypothermia – an update.* Scand. J. Trauma Resus. Emerg. Med. 2016; 24: 111.
4. Gilbert M., Busund R., Skagseth A., Nilsen P.A., Solbø J.P. *Resuscitation from accidental hypothermia of 13.7°C with circulatory arrest.* Lancet 2000; 355(9201): 375–376.
5. Niazi S.A., Lewis F.J. *Profound hypothermia in man; report of a case.* Ann. Surg. 1958; 147(2): 264–266.
6. Castellani J.W., Young A.J. *Human physiological responses to cold exposure: Acute responses and acclimatization to prolonged exposure.* Auton. Neurosci. 2016; 196: 63–74.
7. Zafren K., Giesbrecht G.G., Danzl D.F., Brugger H., Sagalyn E.B., Walpoth B. et al. *Wilderness Medical Society Practice Guidelines for the Out-of-Hospital Evaluation and Treatment of Accidental Hypothermia.* Wilderness Environ. Med. 2014; 25(4): 425–445.
8. Stocks J.M., Taylor N.A.S., Tipton M.J., Greenleaf J.E. *Human physiological responses to cold exposure.* Aviat. Space Environ. Med. 2004; 75: 444–457.
9. Giesbrecht G.G., Bristow G.K., Uin A., Ready A.E., Jones R.A. *Effectiveness of three field treatments for induced mild (33.0°C) hypothermia.* J. Appl. Physiol. 1987; 63: 2375–2379.
10. Eyolfson D., Tikuisis P., Giesbrecht G.G. *Measurement and prediction of maximal shivering capacity in humans.* In: Hodgdon J.A., Heaney J.H., Buono M.J. eds. *Environmental Ergonomics VIII. International Series of Environmental Ergonomics.*

Vol 1. Naval Health Research Center and San Diego State University, San Diego, CA 2000: 315–317.

11. Giesbrecht G.G., Steinman A.M. *Immersion in cold water.* In: Auerbach P.S. ed. *Wilderness Medicine.* 6th ed. Elsevier Mosby, Philadelphia 2012: 143–170.

12. Iampietro P.F., Vaughan J.A., Goldman R.F., Kreider M.B., Masucci F., Bass D.E. *Heat production from shivering.* J. Appl. Physiol. 1960; 15: 632–634.

13. Haman F. *Shivering in the cold: from mechanisms of fuel selection to survival.* J. Appl. Physiol. 2006; 100: 1702–1708.

14. Giesbrecht G.G. *Prehospital treatment of hypothermia.* Wild Environ. Med. 2001; 12: 24–31.

15. Crawshaw L.I., Nagashima K., Yoda T. et al. *Thermoregulation.* In: Auerbach P.S. ed. *Wilderness Medicine.* 6th ed. Mosby Elsevier, Philadelphia, PA 2012: 104–115.

16. Tikuisis P., Ducharme M.B., Moroz D., Jacobs I. *Physiological responses of exercised-fatigued individuals exposed to wet-cold conditions.* J. Appl. Physiol. 1999; 86: 1319–1328.

17. Danzl D.F. *Accidental Hypothermia.* In: Auerbach P.S. ed. *Wilderness Medicine.* 6th ed. Elsevier Mosby, Philadelphia 2012: 116–142.

18. Giesbrecht G.G., Wilkerson J.A. *Too cool to breathe: Evaluation and treatment of hypothermia.* In: Giesbrecht G.G., Wilkerson J.A. eds. *Hypothermia, frostbite and other cold injuries.* The Mountaineers Books, Seattle 2006: 38–56.

19. Oliver S.J., Brierley J.L., Raymond-Barker P.C., Dolci A., Walsh N.P. *Portable prehospital methods to treat near-hypothermic shivering cold casualties.* Wilderness Environ. Med. 2016; 27(1): 125–130.

20. Sran B.J.K., McDonald G.K., Steinman A.M., Gardiner P.F., Giesbrecht G.G. *Comparison of heat donation through the head or torso on mild hypothermia rewarming.* Wild Environ. Med. 2014; 25: 4–13.

21. Giesbrecht G.G., Sessler D.I., Mekjavic I.B., Schroeder M., Bristow G.K. *Treatment of mild immersion hypothermia by direct body-to-body contact.* J. Appl. Physiol. 1994; 76: 2373–2379.

22. Lundgren P., Henriksson O., Naredi P., Bjornstig U. *The effect of active warming in prehospital trauma care during road and air ambulance transportation – a clinical randomized trial.* Scand. J. Trauma Resusc. Emerg. Med. 2011; 19: 59.

23. Lundgren J.P., Henriksson O., Pretorius T., Cahill F., Bristow G., Chochinov A. et al. *Field torso-warming modalities: a comparative study using a human model.* Prehosp. Emerg. Care 2009; 13 (3): 371–378, doi:10.1080/10903120902935348.

24. Williams A.B., Salmon A., Graham P., Galler D., Payton M.J., Bradley M. *Rewarming of healthy volunteers after induced mild hypothermia: a healthy volunteer study.* Emerg. Med. J. 2005; 22(3): 182–184, doi:10.1136/emj.2003.007963.

25. Sterba J.A. *Efficacy and safety of prehospital rewarming techniques to treat accidental hypothermia.* Ann. Emerg. Med. 1991; 20: 896–901.

26. Goheen M.S.L., Ducharme M.B., Kenny G.P., Johnston E., Frim J., Bristow G.K., Gisebrecht G.G. *Efficacy of forced-air and inhalation rewarming by using a human model for severe hypothermia.* J. Appl. Physiol. 1997; 83: 1635–1640.
27. Mekjavić I.B., Eken O. *Inhalation rewarming from hypothermla. An evaluation in –20°C simulated field conditions.* Aviat. Space Environ. Med. 1995; 66: 424–429.
28. Ducharme M.B., Steinman A.M., Giesbrecht G. *Pre-hospital management of immersion hypothermia.* In: Bierens J. ed. *Drowning Prevention, Rescue, Treatment.* 2nd ed. Springer, Berlin 2014: 875–880.
29. Hayward J.S., Eckerson J.D., Kemna D. *Thermal and cardiovascular changes during three methods of resuscitation from mild hypothermia.* Resuscitation 1984; 11: 21–33.
30. Tipton M.J., Ducharme M.B. *Rescue collapse following cold water immersion.* In: Bierens J.J. ed. *Drowning Prevention, Rescue, Treatment.* 2nd ed. Springer, Berlin 2014: 855–858.
31. Golden F.S.C., Hervey G.R. *The "afterdrop" and death after rescue from immersion in cold water.* In: Adam J.A. ed. *Hypothermia ashore and afloat.* Aberdeen University Press, Aberdeen 1981.
32. Giesbrecht G.G. *Cold stress, near drowning and accidental hypothermia: a review.* Aviat. Space Environ. Med. 2000; 71: 733–752.
33. Sultan N., Theakston K.D., Butler R., Suri R.S. *Treatment of severe accidental hypothermia with intermittent hemodialysis.* CJEM 2009; 11: 174–177.
34. Rajek A., Lenhardt R., Sessler D.I. et al. *Tissue heat content and distribution during and after cardiopulmonary bypass at 17°C.* Anesth. Analg. 1999; 88: 1220–1225.
35. Rajek A., Lenhardt R., Sessler D.I. et al. *Efficacy of two methods for reducing post-bypass afterdrop.* Anesthesiology 2000; 92: 447–456.
36. Teodorczyk J.E., Heijmans J.H., van Mook W.N.K.A. et al. *Effectiveness of an underbody forced warm-air blanket during coronary artery bypass surgery in the prevention of postoperative hypothermia: a prospective controlled randomized clinical trial.* Open J. Anesth. 2012; 2: 65–69 (http://dx.doi.org/10.4236/ojanes.2012.23016; accessed: 27.10.2016).
37. Savard G.K., Cooper K.E., Veale W.L., Malkinson T.J. *Peripheral blood flow during rewarming from mild hypothermia in humans.* J. Appl. Physiol. 1985; 58: 4–13.
38. Vanggaard L., Eyolfson D., Xu X. et al. *Immersion of forearms and lower legs in 45°C water effectively rewarms moderately hypothermic subjects.* Aviat. Space Environ. Med. 1999; 11: 1081–1088.
39. Webb P. *Afterdrop of body temperature during rewarming: an alternative explanation.* J. Appl. Physiol. 1986; 60: 385–390.
40. Giesbrecht G.G., Bristow G.K. *The convective afterdrop component during hypothermic exercise decreases with delayed exercise onset.* Aviat. Space Environ. Med. 1998; 69(1): 17–22.
41. Giesbrecht G.G., Bristow G.K. *A second postcooling afterdrop: more evidence for a convective mechanism.* J. Appl. Physiol. 1992; 73(4): 1253–1258.

42. Giesbrecht G.G., Goheen M.S., Johnston C.E., Kenny G.P., Bristow G.K., Hayward J.S. *Inhibition of shivering increases core temperature afterdrop and attenuates rewarming in hypothermic humans.* J. Appl. Physiol. 1997; 83(5): 1630–1634.

43. Hultzer M., Xu X., Marrao C., Bristow G.K., Chochinov A., Giesbrecht G.G. *Pre-hospital torso-warmingmodalities for severe hypothermia: a comparative study using a human model.* Can. J. Emerg. Med. 2005; 7: 378–386.

44. Miles J.M., Thompson G.R. *Treatment of severe accidental hypothermia using the Clinitron bed.* Anaesthesia 1987; 42: 415–418.

45. Koller R., Schnider T.W., Neidhart P. *Deep accidental rewarming with hypothermia and cardiac arrest – forced air.* Acta Anaes. Scand. 1997; 41: 1359–1364.

46. Steele M.T., Nelson M.J., Sessler D.I., Fraker L., Bunney B., Watson W.A., Robinson W.A. *Forced air speeds rewarming in accidental hypothermia.* Ann. Emerg. Med. 1996; 27: 479–484.

47. Bräuer A., Wrigge H., Kersten J., Rathgeber J., Weyland W., Burchardi H. *Severe accidental hypothermia: rewarming strategy using a veno-venous bypass system and a convective air warmer.* Int. Care Med. 1999; 25: 520–523.

48. Kornberger E., Schwarz B., Lindner K.H., Mair P. *Forced air surface rewarming in patients with severe accidental hypothermia.* Resuscitation 1999; 41: 105–111.

49. Greif R., Rajek A., Laciny S., Bastanmehr H., Sessler D. *Resistive heating is more effective than metallic-foil insulation in an experimental model of accidental hypothermia: a randomized controlled trial.* Ann. Emerg. Med. 2000; 35: 337–345.

50. Willekes T., Naunheim R., Lasater M. *A novel method of intravascular temperature modulation to treat severe hypothermia.* Emerg. Med. J. 2006; 23(10): e56, doi:10.1136/emj.2006.035360.

51. Caluwé R., Vanholder R., Dhondt A. *Hemodialysis as a treatment of severe accidental hypothermia.* Artif. Org. 2010; 34: 237–239.

52. Cocchi M.N., Giberson B., Donnino M.W. *Rapid rewarming of hypothermic patient using Arctic Sun device.* J. Int. Care Med. 2012; 27: 128–130.

53. Brown D., Ellerton J., Paal P., Boyd J. *Hypothermia Evidence, Afterdrop and Practical Experience.* Wilderness Environ. Med. 2015; 26(3): 437–439.

54. Zafren K., Giesbrecht G.G., Danzl D.F., Brugger H., Sagalyn E.B., Walpoth B. et al. *Hypothermia Evidence, Afterdrop, and Guidelines.* Wilderness Environ. Med. 2015; 26(3): 439–441.

55. Covino B.G., Beavers W.R. *Effect of hypothermia on ventricular fibrillary threshold.* Exp. Biol. Med. 1957; 95: 631–634.

56. Mortensen E., Bernsten R., Tveita T., Lathrop D.A., Refsum H. *Changes in ventricular fibrillation threshold during acute hypothermia: a model for future studies.* J. Basic Clin. Physiol. 1993, doi: 10.1515/JBCPP.1993.4.4.313.

57. Brugger H., Paal P., Boyd J. *Prehospital resuscitation of the buried avalanche victim.* High Alt. Med. Biol. 2011; 12: 199–205.

58. Roberts D.E., Barr J.C., Kerr D. et al. *Fluid replacement during hypothermia*. Aviat. Space Environ. Med. 1985; 56: 333–337.

59. Thomassen O., Færevik H., Østerås O., Sunde G.A., Zakariassen E., Sandsund M. et al. *Comparison of three different prehospital wrapping methods for preventing hypothermia – a crossover study in humans*. Scand. J. Trauma Resusc. Emerg. Med. 2011; 19: 41, doi:10.1186/1757-7241-19-41.

60. Henriksson O., Lundgren P., Kuklane K., Holmer I., Naredi P., Bjornstig U. *Protection against cold in prehospital care: evaporative heat loss reduction by wet clothing removal or the addition of a vapor barrier-a thermal manikin study*. Prehosp. Disaster Med. 2012; 27(1): 53–58, doi:10.1017/S1049023X12000210.

61. Henriksson O., Lundgren P.J., Kuklane K., Holmer I., Giesbrecht G.G., Naredi P. et al. *Protection against cold in prehospital care: wet clothing removal or addition of a vapor barrier*. Wilderness Environ. Med. 2015; 26(1): 11–20, doi:10.1016/j.wem.2014.07.001.

62. Henriksson O., Lundgren P., Kuklane K., Holmér I., Bjornstig U. *Protection against cold in prehospital care – thermal insulation properties of blankets and rescue bags in different wind conditions*. Prehosp. Disaster Med. 2009; 24: 408–415.

63. Golden F., Tipton M.J. *Castaways: survival in an open boat or life craft*. In: Golden F.T.M. ed. *Essentials of Sea Survival*. Edn. Human Kinetics, Leeds 2002: 177–213.

64. Brugger H., Procter E., Rauch S., Strapazzon G. *Cooling rate for triage decisions should exclude post-extrication cooling in avalanche victims*. Resuscitation 2015; 94: e3, doi:10.1016/j.resuscitation.2015.06.020.

65. House J., Fleming M., Tipton M. *Incorporating water absorbent and reflective layers into a survival bag does not improve temperature recovery of cold wet humans*. XIV International Conference on Environmental Ergonomics, Greece 2011.

66. Chadwick S., Gibson A. *Hypothermia and the use of space blankets: a literature review*. Accid. Emerg. Nurs. 1997; 5: 122–125.

67. *Metallized plastic sheeting for use in cold climate survival*. Alpine J. 1977; 82: 126.

68. Zasa M., Flowers N., Zideman D., Hodgetts T.J., Harris T. *A torso model comparison of temperature preservation devices for use in the prehospital environment*. Emerg. Med. J. 2016; 33(6): 418–422, doi:10.1136/emermed-2015-204769.

69. Jussila K., Rissanen S., Parkkola K., Anttonen H. *Evaluating cold, wind, and moisture protection of different coverings for prehospital maritime transportation-a thermal manikin and human study*. Prehosp. Disaster Med. 2014; 29(6): 580–588, doi:10.1017/S1049023X14001125.

70. Thomassen O., Østerås O., Brattebø G., Karlsen A., Gløersen J. *A non evaporation layer combined with insulation is the preferred method for prevention of prehospital hypothermia*. Eur. J. Anaes. 2010; 27: 190 (Abstr. 13AP1-5).

71. Truhlár A., Deakin C.D., Soar J., Khalifa G.E., Alfonzo A., Bierens J.J. et al. *European Resuscitation Council Guidelines for Resuscitation 2015: Section 4. Cardiac*

arrest in special circumstances. Resuscitation 2015; 95: 148–201, doi:10.1016/j. resuscitation.2015.07.017.

72. Watts D.D., Roche M., Tricarico R., Poole F., Brown J.J., Colson G.B., Trask A.L., Fakhry S.M. *The utility of traditional prehospital interventions in maintaining thermostasis*. Prehosp. Emerg. Care 1999; 3: 115–122.

73. Giesbrecht G.G., Pachu P., Xu X. *Design and evaluation of a portable rigid forced-air warming cover for prehospital transport of cold patients*. Aviat. Space Environ. Med. 1998; 69: 1200–1203.

74. Ostertag H., Hibler H. *General hypothermia. First aid and clinical treatment*. Fortschritte der Medizin 1981; 99(19): 707–711 (Abstract only available).

75. Ennemoser O., Ambach W., Flora G. *Physical assessment of heat insulation rescue foils*. Int. J. Sports Med. 1988; 9: 179–182.

76. Paal P., Beikircher W., Brugger H. *Der Lawinennotfall*. Der Anaesthetist 2006; 55: 314–324.

77. Owen R., Castle N. *Prehospital temperature control*. Emerg. Med. J. 2008; 25: 375–376, doi:10.1136/emj.2008.059030.

14

Coagulopathies in Hypothermic Patient

Hubert Hymczak[1], Mirosław Ziętkiewicz[2,3], Dariusz Plicner[4]

[1] Severe Hypothermia Treatment Centre, Department of Anaesthesiology and Intensive Care, John Paul II Hospital, Cracow, Poland
[2] Department of Anaesthesiology and Pulmonary Intensive Care, John Paul II Hospital, Cracow, Poland
[3] Chair of Anaesthesiology and Intensive Care, Jagiellonian University Collegium Medicum, Cracow, Poland
[4] The Department of Cardiovascular Surgery and Transplantation, John Paul II Hospital, Cracow, Poland

Pathophysiology

Haemostasis is a group of complex and inter-related processes maintaining integrity of blood vessels both in normal conditions as well as after vessel damage. The role of haemostasis in case of vessel wall damage is formation of clot, followed by fibrinolysis and restoration of normal flow.

Proper functioning of haemostasis is enabled by plasma components, mainly platelets, blood vessel wall (vascular endothelium), as well as coagulation and fibrinolysis systems. In normal conditions, balance between coagulation and fibrinolysis systems is maintained.

Coagulation system, particularly in its plasmatic aspect, is a series of enzymatic reactions vitally dependent on temperature and pH. The optimal functioning of the system coincides with physiological body temperature, hence drop in body temperature entails significant disturbances in the process.

Coagulopathy in hypothermia is a result of decrease in activity number of platelets, reduction in activity of plasma coagulation factors, and enzymatic processes [1–3]. Relationship between drop in blood temperature and occurrence of coagulopathy, however, is not linear. It is accepted that decrease of 1°C of body temperature causes decrease of function of coagulation system by 10%.

Hypothermia in the range 37–33°C causes mainly platelets adhesion disorders without disturbing significantly neither their activation nor enzymatic activity of plasma factors [1–4]. Furthermore, an increased sensitivity of blood platelets to pro-coagulation factors is observed, what translates into increased capacity to form clots in peripheral parts of the body, more exposed to potential injury [4]. Only in temperature lower than 33°C significant haemostasis disorders are observed, related mainly to reduced activity of thrombocytes and enzymatic activity [1, 2, 5].

Paradoxically, in chronic hypothermia (with polyuria and dehydration) haemoconcentration with increase of hematocrit by 2% for each °C < 34°C may occur [6, 7], as well as vasoconstriction, release of tissue thromboplastins, and increase in fibrinogen concentration. These may lead to clotting and occurrence of embolism.

Progressive thrombocytopenia occurs usually below 30°C. It is caused by increased capture of thrombocytes, mainly by liver and spleen, and their so called margination (shift to perimeter of the vessel), their change in shape, decrease in speed of blood flow, and increase in expression of adhesion molecules [1, 3, 5]. Despite the drop in temperature, capacity of platelets to activate is not obliterated, as opposed to their adhesion and aggregation capabilities, which are reduced [3].

In progressed hypothermia (below 33–34°C), activity and number of plasma coagulation factors become reduced, thrombin production is also decreased [8–10]. It is believed that this process is the main reason behind coagulopathy in hypothermia.

Early stages of hypothermia affect fibrinolysis system only slightly. Only after drop of temperature to below 20°C fibrinolysis system undergoes strong activation [1]. Drop of body temperature to below 16°C deactivates coagulation system almost entirely without affecting the already formed clots.

Post-traumatic hypothermia

Hypothermia is also an important factor leading to post-traumatic coagulation disorders (Acute Traumatic Coagulopathy), which correlates with worse prognosis and increased post traumatic fatality [11, 12]. Hypothermia together with metabolic acidosis and coagulopathy are labelled as "lethal triad" in traumatic patients [2, 12]. Post-traumatic hypothermia has been described in detail in Chapter 11. It is worth noting that one of the main risk factors of hypothermia and post-traumatic coagulopathy is excessive intravenous fluid therapy (both with crystalloids as well as colloids) administered in order to maintain perfusion pressure [2, 8, 13, 14]. The negative impact of crystalloid infusions results mainly from blood dilution. Colloid solutions additionally disturb fibrin polymerisation, reduce elasticity, and size of clot. In combination with crystalloids, colloids may cause drop in von Willebrand factor concentration. Hydroxyethyl starch solutions may increase risk of bleeding, leading to hypocalcaemia, platelets, fibrinogen, and von Willebrand factor disorders as well as disturbances in fibrin polymerisation process.

Diagnostics

Laboratory diagnostic of coagulation system in hypothermic patients is significantly hindered. The reason for this is the standard procedure to perform tests at 37°C. Plasmatic and platelets function parameters measured in such a fashion may present results in normal ranges, whilst in reality coagulation is severely disturbed. Hypothermia prolongs prothrombin and partial thromboplastin times proportionately to drop in temperature [8, 15]. Determining *in vitro* coagulation times in lower temperature causes their additional prolonging in comparison to measurements obtained from the same sample in 37°C [2, 16]. Thrombocytopenia, as mentioned before, is caused mainly by redistribution, so it is merely ostensible.

The only efficient method of evaluation of coagulation system in entirety is thromboelastography (TEG). TEG determines the process of formation and degradation of clot in full blood in a simple and clear manner.

A single test encompasses both cellular, enzymatic, and coagulation factors as well as fibrinolysis process. One of the important advantages of TEG is a possibility to calibrate to patient's body temperature [1, 12, 13, 16, 17]. Despite the unequivocal diagnostic value of the test it is rarely available in Polish hospitals.

Therapy

Rewarming the patient to normothermia causes gradual return of plasma coagulation factors activity and normalisation of number and function of thrombocytes – more than 80% of captured platelets may return to circulation after release from liver and spleen.

    Any interference in haemostasis before rewarming may be very hazardous. Transfusions of plasma, coagulation factors concentrate, or platelets concentrate performed upon tests results and without clinical examination are pointless, as each of these blood products becomes "inactivated" by low temperature, and after rewarming may become a reason for hypercoagulability with all grave consequences.

Haemostatic resuscitation

In accidental post-exposure hypothermia, haemostatic resuscitation is indicated only exceptionally, but it is usually necessary in post-traumatic hypothermia. In patients with massive haemorrhage and signs of coagulopathy it is recommended to perform early transfusions of packed red blood cells, platelets concentrate, and fresh frozen plasma according to 1:1:1 ratio [12, 14].

    After achieving normothermia, in presence of continuing haemorrhage and laboratory test confirmed haemostasis disorders, substitution of lacking factors and optionally of antyfibrinolitic substances may be indicated [8, 10, 12, 14, 18–20]:

- Fibrinogen, cryoprecipitate – in decrease in plasma below 1,0 g/dL. It is worth keeping in mind that in severe blood loss fibrinogen level reaches critical values before other pro-coagulation factors and platelets reach minimal values.

- Recombinant active factor VII – forms a complex with tissue factor and phospholipids in place of vessel damage, transforming factor X into Xa and factor IX into IXa, activates coagulation system and promotes local haemostasis. Factor VIIa activates also factor X on the surface of activated platelets in place of damage independently from tissue factor. Its use is associated with possible risk of DIC (disseminated intravascular coagulation), moreover it is not registered for use in bleeding resulting from trauma (it is an off-label use).
- Prothrombin complex concentrate (PCC) – obtained from human plasma, contains 2530 times more coagulation factors than fresh frozen plasma, its use carries no risk of volume overload. Currently European guidelines recommend its use only in urgent cases with goal of reversal of vitamin K antagonists.
- Tranexamic acid – an anti-fibrinolytic agent with proven efficacy in mortality reduction in early use in heamorrhage [20].

It should be emphasised that rewarming process is associated with risk of occurrence of DIC [3, 15, 20]. As opposed to reduced activity of coagulation system and increased fibrinolysis in course of hypothermia, DIC in early phase is a condition of increased activity of coagulation system. Vast prothrombotic activation in DIC may lead to coagulopathy by exhaustion of clotting factors. Diagnosis is based on clinical signs, including internal organs damage and laboratory tests. Treatment initially involves stabilisation of general condition, and subsequently halting overstimulated coagulation process and restoring insufficiencies of haemostasis system to norm [2, 18].

Summary

Disorders of coagulation system in hypothermic patient are difficult to detect with laboratory tests. Coagulopathy aggravates with drop of body temperature and is alleviated by rewarming. Treatment thus should primarily involve treatment of causes, i.e. efficient rewarming, which in most cases restores haemostasis to norm. Substitutional treatment may be indicated only in massive haemorrhage. It should be remembered that occurrence of DIC is possible on every phase of therapy.

References

1. Brinkman A.C., Ten Tusscher B.L., de Waard M.C. et al. *Minimal effects on ex vivo coagulation during mild therapeutic hypothermia in post cardiac arrest patients.* Resuscitation 2014; 85(10): 1359–1363.
2. Palmer L., Martin L. *Traumatic coagulopathy – part 1: Pathophysiology and diagnosis.* J. Vet. Emerg. Crit. Care (San Antonio) 2014; 24(1): 63–74.
3. Weidman J.L., Shook D.C., Hilberath J.N. *Cardiac resuscitation and coagulation.* Anesthesiology 2014; 120(4): 1009–1014.
4. Egidi M.G., D'Alessandro A., Mandarello G. et al. *Troubleshooting in platelet storage temperature and new perspectives through proteomics.* Blood Transfus. 2010; 8(Suppl. 3): 73–81.
5. Winokur R., Hartwig J.H. *Mechanism of shape change in chilled human platelets.* Blood 1995; 85: 1796–1804.
6. Sosnowski P., Mikrut K., Krauss H. *Hypothermia – mechanism of action and pathophysiological changes in the human body.* Postępy Hig. Med. Dosw. 2015; 69: 69–79.
7. Danzl D.F., Pozos S.R. *Accidental hypothermia.* N. Engl. J. Med. 1994; 331: 1756–1760.
8. Schlimp C.J., Schöchl H. *The role of fibrinogen in trauma-induced coagulopathy.* Hamostaseologie 2014; 34(1): 29–39.
9. Mitrophanov A.Y., Rosendaal F.R., Reifman J. *Computational analysis of the effects of reduced temperature on thrombin generation: the contributions of hypothermia to coagulopathy.* Anesth. Analg. 2013; 117(3): 565–574.
10. Maung A.A., Kaplan L.J. *Role of fibrinogen in massive injury.* Minerva Anestesiol. 2014; 80(1): 89–95.
11. Davenport R. *Pathogenesis of acute traumatic coagulopathy.* Transfusion 2013; 53: 23S–27S.
12. Simmons J.W., Pittet J.F., Pierce B. *Trauma-Induced Coagulopathy.* Curr. Anesthesiol. Rep. 2014; 4(3): 189–199.
13. Katrancha E.D., Gonzalez L.S. 3rd. *Trauma-induced coagulopathy.* Crit. Care Nurse 2014; 34(4): 54–63.
14. Christiaans S.C., Duhachek-Stapelman A.L., Russell R.T. et al. *Coagulopathy after severe pediatric trauma.* Shock 2014; 41(6): 476–490.
15. Mahajan S.L., Myers T.J., Baldini M.G. *Disseminated intravascular coagulation during rewarming following hypothermia.* JAMA 1981; 245: 2517–1518.

16. Forman K.R., Wong E., Gallagher M. et al. *Effect of temperature on thromboelastography and implications for clinical use in newborns undergoing therapeutic hypothermia.* Pediatr. Res. 2014; 75(5): 663–669.
17. Kander T., Brokopp J., Friberg H. et al. *Wide temperature range testing with ROTEM coagulation analyses.* Ther. Hypothermia Temp. Manag. 2014; 4(3): 125–130.
18. Cap A., Hunt B.J. *The pathogenesis of traumatic coagulopathy.* Anaesthesia 2015; 70(Suppl. 1): 96–101, e32–e34.
19. Palmer L., Martin L. *Traumatic coagulopathy – part 2: Resuscitative strategies.* J. Vet. Emerg. Crit. Care (San Antonio) 2014; 24(1): 75–92.
20. Roberts I., Shakur H., Coats T. et al. *The CRASH-2 trial: a randomised controlled trial and economic evaluation of the effects of tranexamic acid on death, vascular occlusive events and transfusion requirement in bleeding trauma patients.* Health Technol. Assess. 2013; 17(10): 1–79.

15

Changes of Pharmacokinetics and Pharmacodynamics of Medications in Hypothermic Patients

Jarosław Woroń[1,2], Jerzy Wordliczek[1]

[1] Anaesthesiology and Intensive Care Unit no. 1, Emergency and Mass-Event Medicine Trauma Centre, The University Hospital in Cracow, Poland
[2] Chair of Pharmacology, Jagiellonian University Collegium Medicum, Cracow, Poland

Medications administered to human organism undergo various subsequent pharmacokinetic processes. The drug must, first of all, be released from its formulation, i.e. tablet, capsule or suppository etc. Next, it is absorbed from various areas depending on the administration route – gastrointestinal tract when administered orally or rectally, subcutaneous or muscular tissue when given in form of tissue injection. Medications can be also absorbed through skin, and various types of mucous membrane other than in GI tract, e.g. in vagina or conjunctival sac of the eye. Volatile liquids, gasses and fine particles of solid bodies administered as aerosols or fine colloids can be absorbed by the lungs. Only drugs administered directly to circulatory system (intravenously, intra-arterially) are distributed instantaneously after administration, without release and absorption processes [1]. Both absorption as well as permeation of medications to tissues relies on transportation through various biological membranes. Such modes of transportation are: simple diffusion, convective transport, carrier mediated transport (facilitated diffusion and active transport), and pinocytosis. The essential role is played by simple diffusion and active transport. Simple diffusion is permeation of non-ionized and lipid-soluble particles through lipid membrane

– the process is a movement down concentration gradient, is non-competitive and does not become saturated. Active transport is enabled by carrier system in cell membrane – the movement is against concentration gradient, is energy-dependent and its maximal speed is limited by number of carrier particles, it is competitively inhibited. Most of the processes described are determined in assumed physiological conditions [1].

One of the significant parameters capable of altering drugs efficacy is body temperature. In pharmacokinetics pertaining to physiological state, speed of processes is evaluated in normothermia (36–37°C) [1]. Hypothermia and hyperthermia may cause alterations in distribution, metabolism, and elimination processes of a drug, what in clinical practice translates into variation in response to administered drug, frequently a necessity to modify doses, and different profile of potential side effects. Majority of medications after reaching circulatory system become bound to blood proteins – protein-bound drug is inactive, does not become distributed, biotransformed, or excreted. In hypothermic patients binding to proteins may occur to a lower extent what implies a larger fraction of free drug i.e. available for receptors in target tissues [1, 2].

The effect of a drug is its ability to permeate to tissues, particularly to target tissue/organ. Drugs crossing the blood-brain barrier and into central nervous system as well as permeating through placenta to foetus are of special importance [1–3].

Most of drugs undergo biotransformation which transforms lipophilic and apolar substances into hydrophilic and polar ones, as only in this form they may be excreted by kidneys – the main route of excretion of majority of drugs. Biotransformation, occurring mainly in liver, usually causes the loss of pharmacological effect of the drug. Activity of enzymes taking part in biotransformation depends on species, sex (most of drugs are metabolised faster in males), age, physiological condition, body temperature, ambient temperature, illness and presence of enzyme inhibitors, which inhibit biotransformation of drugs, as well as enzyme inducers, which intensify biotransformation. Some medications, e.g. barbiturates or morphine, posses capability to auto-induce, i.e. to increase rate of their own metabolism, what is the reason behind development of tolerance to those drugs [1, 3].

Drugs are removed from the organism via kidneys with urine, via liver with bile, to a smaller degree with spit, by intestines, lungs (volatile compounds) or by skin with sweat. Renal excretion of drugs may occur as filtration through pores in the glomerular endothelium and as selective elimination in renal tubules. Glomerular excretion involves only the fraction of the drug that is not protein bound. Intensity of this elimination process depends on renal blood flow and permeability of glomeruli. Renal ducts excretion, on the other hand, is an active transport of certain substances to urine. Both efficacy of glomerular excretion as well as duct excretion of drugs can become diminished in hypothermic patients, and magnitude of diminishment is proportional to decrease in body temperature [1–3].

In hypothermic patients diminishment of bioavailability is also likely, which is defined as fraction of drug accessing systemic circulation from the place of administration. It is not synonymous with absorption, as after absorption in e.g. intestine some drugs undergo a process of first--pass: a portion of drug is metabolised in intestinal wall or liver. Bioavailability of a given formulation of a drug determines its blood serum concentration, thus its effect. In hypothermic patients oral and rectal drug administration routes are not recommended as the effects of drugs administered via these routes are difficult to predict.

After absorption into blood, drug concentration decreases. Most often (if it is a phase I process) the concentration of a drug in a period of time decreases proportionally – i.e. if after an hour it drops by 10%, in each following hour it will be dropping by the same percentage. The numerical value of this process is elimination constant. The opposite of elimination constant is elimination half-life, i.e. the time required for the concentration of the drug to reach half of its original value. So, if a half-life of a drug is 1 hour, its concentration will decrease by half every hour. Elimination constant and elimination half- life are not fixed values – they change depending on dose of drug, among other factors. Elimination half life depends on individual characteristics, genotype, nutrition, recreational drugs intake, life-style, age and body temperature. Changes in pharmacokinetics of drugs, their degree and clinical importance are related to severity of hypothermia. More significant changes are observable in moderate stage (28–32°C) than in mild (33–35°C) [1–4].

In hypothermic patients activity of cytochrome P450 isoenzymes changes, what is particularly important when administering drugs actively metabolised by these isoenzymes. Such changes are clearly visible in patients with varying pharmacokinetics of medications. These include:

newborns, children up to age of 12, and patients above 65 years of age. Isoenzyme CYP3A4 metabolises more than 50% of all drugs used in pharmacotherapy. It partakes, among others, in metabolism of midazolam and other medications used in intensive care. Drugs metabolised by CYP3A4, whose metabolism may change in hypothermia, were summarised in Table 1 [1, 2, 5, 6].

Table 1. Drugs metabolised by CYP3A4, whose metabolism may change in hypothermia

amiodarone
amlodipine
ciprofloxacin
dexamethasone
haloperidol
lignocaine
prednisone
theophylline
valproic acid

Source: Authors' own compilation.

Hypothermia may also alter metabolism of drugs metabolised with CYP2C9 and CYP2C19 isoenzymes. This pertains particularly to propranolol, omeprazole, and diazepam, doses of these drugs should be reduced by about 20–30% [2, 4, 5, 7].

Isoenzyme CYP2D6 partakes in metabolism of 25% of commonly used medications. It is worth remembering that about 7–10% of members of Polish population metabolise substrates of CYP2D6 slowly, and this effect can be aggravated by hypothermia. Special attention should be given to patients whom metoprolol and rocuronium are administered, the doses of these drugs should be adjusted individually according to desired pharmacologic effect. In hypothermia also drug conjugation processes occurring in liver become diminished, what may result in increased concentration of certain drugs in plasma. An example is morphine, whose concentration in plasma tends to increase, so the dose should be reduced [1, 2, 4, 7].

Table 2 summarises information concerning effect of hypothermia onto pharmacokinetics of medications used in intensive care, along with clinical consequences of these effects [2, 4, 5, 7].

Table 2. Hypothermia vs pharmacokinetics of drugs

Drug	Effect of hypothermia	Consequences for drug use
remifentanyl fentanyl	clearance reduction drop in distribution volume	reduction of dose by about 30%
morphine	increased blood plasma concentration prolonged half-life	reduction of dose by about 30% slower titration of dose
propofol	increased blood plasma concentration	reduction of dose by about 30%
midazolam	increased blood plasma concentration rise in distribution volume	reduction of dose depending on pharmacological effect
vecuronium rocuronium	clearance reduction prolonged time to beginning of pharmacological effect	reduction of dose by about 30%
atracurium	clearance reduction	delay of intubation
glyceryl trinitrate	clearance reduction	reduction of dose depending on pharmacological effect
phenytoin	clearance reduction reduced concentration of both blod protein bound as well as of free fraction	reduction of dose depending on pharmacological effect

Source: Own compiled upon Tortorici M.A., Kochanek P.M., Poloyac S.M. *Effects of hypothermia on drug disposition, metabolism and response.* Crit. Care Med. 2007; 35: 2196–2204 [2]; Bauer L.A. *Applied Clinical Pharmacokinetics.* McGraw-Hill Education, New York 2014 [4]; Zhou J., Poloyac S.M. *The effect of therapeutic hypothermia on drug metabolism and drug response.* Expert Opin. Drug Metab. Toxicol. 2011; 7: 803–816 [5]; van den Broek M.P.H., Groenendaal F., Egberts A.C.G. et al. *Effects of hypothermia on pharmacokinetics and pharmacodynamics.* Clin. Pharmacokinet. 2010; 49: 277–294 [7].

Electrolyte disorders are often met in hypothermic patients – if hypokalaemia, hypomagnesaemia or hypophosphataemia occur, the change of anti-arrhythmic drugs effect also takes place. Special caution should thus be kept together with constant ECG monitoring in patients who receive QT interval prolonging medication. Hypokalaemia and hypomagnesaemia favour occurence of the most dangerous clinical effect of QT prolonging, namely *torsade de pointes* [4, 7].

In hypothermia, the processes of diffusion of drugs via biological membranes do not become significantly altered, yet active transport can be distorted. As a consequence, changes of therapeutic outcome of digoxin and verapamil administration may be observed [4, 7].

Hypothermia affects also drug elimination process – usually glomerular filtration becomes reduced. It is worth remembering that in hypothermia synthesis of creatinine is diminished, what causes limited use of monitoring of creatinine clearance as a measurement of renal filtration rate.

Increasingly more numerous clinical studies provide new data on changes of pharmacokinetics of drugs in hypothermic patients. Most of the data allows for direct conclusions for clinical practice, however, the individual, patient-dependent factors which may affect the final outcome of pharmacotherapy should not be forgotten. Further observations will allow for broadening the practical knowledge on this subject [2, 4, 7].

References

1. DiPiro J.T., Talbert L.R., Yee G.C. et al. *Pharmacotherapy, a pathophysiologic approach*. McGraw-Hill Education, New York 2014.
2. Tortorici M.A., Kochanek P.M., Poloyac S.M. *Effects of hypothermia on drug disposition, metabolism and response*. Crit. Care Med. 2007; 35: 2196–2204.
3. Kaye A.D., Kaye A.M., Urman R.D. *Essentials of Pharmacology for Anaesthesia, Pain Medicine and Critical Care*. Springer, New York 2015.
4. Bauer L.A. *Applied Clinical Pharmacokinetics*. McGraw-Hill Education, New York 2014.
5. Zhou J., Poloyac S.M. *The effect of therapeutic hypothermia on drug metabolism and drug response*. Expert Opin. Drug Metab. Toxicol. 2011; 7: 803–816.
6. Kostka-Trąbka E., Woroń J. *Interakcje leków w praktyce klinicznej*. Wydawnictwo Lekarskie PZWL, Warszawa 2011.
7. van den Broek M.P.H., Groenendaal F., Egberts A.C.G. i in. *Effects of hypothermia on pharmacokinetics and pharmacodynamics*. Clin. Pharmacokinet. 2010; 49: 277–294.

16

Extracorporeal Therapy in Patients in Severe Hypothermia

Rafał Drwiła

Department of Anaesthesiology and Intensive Care, John Paul II Hospital, Cracow, Poland
Chair of Anaesthesiology and Intensive Care, Jagiellonian University Collegium Medicum, Cracow, Poland

Introduction

Fast pace of technology advancement, which has been observed since the beginning of 21st century, gives at the disposal of therapeutic teams possibilities which had been practiced priorly only in selected, highly specialised medical centres. Exhaustion of pharmacological means of treatment of acute and end-stage circulatory failure has pointed the attention of the researchers to use of mechanical support and replacement of heart function also outside of specialised cardiac surgery centres, i.e. in other medical facilities, such as emergency care wards. System of extracorporeal membrane oxygenation (ECMO) is currently implemented for various indications.

The most important of them are:

- cardiac indications resulting from myocardial heart failure;
- pulmonary indications resulting from pulmonary failure;
- other indications (severe hypothermia, poisonings, septic shock et al.);
- organ transplantation indications (support of organs functions).

In this paper I would like to present basic ECMO principles and uses, along with applications in emergency care.

History of ECMO use

The first application of extracorporeal circulation during cardiac surgery was described by Gibbon in 1953. Unfortunately, the device used then was unable to operate for longer than 6 hours. In 1971 Hill reported on three-day-long treatment of a patient in acute respiratory distress syndrome (ARDS), what made the method popular in treatment of patients with lung damage. The genuine breakthrough in extracorporeal blood oxygenation was the establishment of Extracorporeal Life Support Organization (ELSO) in New Orleans, monitoring and coordinating the development of this method in various medical centres. Large multi-centre, randomised trial (CESAR), published in 2009, has shown a substantial reduction of fatality rate among patients with ARDS treated with ECMO in veno-venous configuration. H1N1 influenza pandemic has made medical professionals and decision-makers aware of the necessity to further develop the technology. ECMO in veno-arterial configuration is currently used for treatment of circulatory failure of different aetiology. It should be remembered that the usage of ECMO is practiced in a patient group distinguished by almost 100% fatality rate. According to ELSO report the number of ECMO usages in almost 300 centres cooperating with the organisation has exceeded 50,000 in 2012.

Basic principles of ECMO functioning

Despite the complicated appearance of ECMO device, the principle of it functioning is relatively simple. At the beginning it should be stated that ECMO system is a closed one, with no direct contact between oxygen and air blend and blood of the patient. Internal surface of the apparatus is coated with glycoproteins or heparin derivatives, what reduces inflammatory response and facilitates anti-coagulative measures taken during the treatment.

The heart of the apparatus is naturally a pump enabling the blood flow (Figure 1). In the early versions of ECMO it was a roller pump used widely in extracorporeal circulation devices. The damage of blood cells was a main factor limiting the runtime of the device. Introduction of routine use of centrifugal pumps, where blood flow is enabled by vanes rotating in electromagnetic field, has made possible prolonging of the device runtime even up to several weeks. One should of course keep in mind the non-occlusive pump operation characteristic, what makes permanent control of the flow by means of electromagnetic and ultrasonographic sensors necessary. Blood flow achieved by means of centrifugal pump usually does not exceed 7 litres per minute.

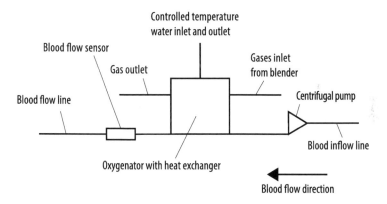

Figure 1. Schematic representation of ECMO device

Source: Author's own compilation.

Another important element of the system is the oxygenator responsible for elimination of carbon dioxide produced in the organism and supply of oxygen indispensable for metabolic processes (Figure 2). The characteristics of commonly used oxygenators are listed in Table 1.

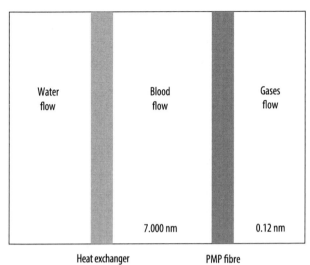

Figure 2. Cross-section through commonly used oxygenators

Source: Author's own compilation.

Table 1. Characteristics of oxygenators

Oxygenator properties	Sorin EOS ECMO	Maquet Quadrox PLS	Maquet HLS Module Integrated Centrifugal Pump	Medos Hilite 7000 LT
blood flow rate	0.5–5 L/min	0.5–7 L/min	0.5–7 L/min	0–7 L/min
membrane surface area	1.2 m²	1.8 m²	1.8 m²	1.9 m²
membrane type	PMP fibre	PMP fibre	PMP fibre	PMP fibre
biomedical coating	phosphorylcho- line	bioline	bioline	rheoparin
fill volume	150 ml	250 ml	273 ml	270 ml
heat exchanger surface area	0.14 m²	0.6 m²	0.4 m²	0.45 m²
heat exchanger area	stainless steel	polyurethane	polyurethane	polyesther

Source: Author's own compilation.

Gas exchange surface area of the most popular oxygenators ranges from 1.2 to 1.9 m². The most often used material is polymethylpentene (PMP), whose structure enables easy gas exchange and simultaneously makes escape of plasma through membrane impossible. Delivery of air-oxygen blend from a container directly into oxygenator gas compartment necessitates removal of carbon dioxide and diffusion of oxygen to blood in accordance with pressure gradient (Figure 2). One must not forget that contemporary oxygenators are equipped with heat exchanger characterised by exchange surface area of 0.14 to 0.6 m², in which water is used as heat carrier. This in particular enables warming of the flowing blood.

Gas exchange in oxygenator depends on various factors. Elimination of carbon dioxide is possible already in lower blood flow rates (1.5 litre per minute), what stems from physical and chemical properties of CO_2. Full oxygenation of the patient whose lungs are entirely incapacitated is possible in blood flow rates comparable to physiological (Figure 3). A persistent issue is a decrease in gas exchange rate observed during oxygenator operation. Currently used devices should not operate for longer than 14 days. When prolonged runtimes are necessary the devices can be exchanged by the patient's bed with ease. Not observing the anticoagulation recommendations typically listed in oxygenator characteristics, usually results in fast drop of the device's efficacy and necessitates replacement.

Currently used heat exchangers enable relatively fast change of patient's core temperature. During rewarming it should be kept in mind that temperature increase rate should be maintained within the rage of 4–6°C per hour and maximum gradient of 10°C between warming water and patient's blood. Not following these guidelines may precipitate severe neurological complications and haemolisys.

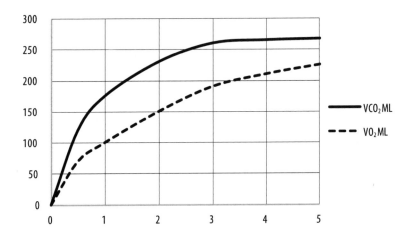

Figure 3. Relationship between blood flow (horizontal axis, in L/min) and gas exchange (vertical axis, in mL/min). **ML** – carbon dioxide flow in mL/min. VO_2ML – flow of oxygen in mL/min

Source: Author's own research.

The third component of ECMO system is set of cannulas receiving the blood of the patient, returning the blood to the patient along with tubing integrating the whole system. Depending on configuration of receiving and returning cannulas ECMO systems can be categorised in two groups:

- V-A ECMO – when the blood is withdrawn from the venous system and returned to arterial system (Figure 4);
- V-V ECMO – when the blood is withdrawn from the venous system and returned to venous system (Figure 5).

Choice of cannulation method depends on myocardium efficiency. In case of abnormalities in myocardium functioning the kinetic energy transferred to oxygenated blood transfused to arterial system in V-A ECMO configuration provides mechanical support of both circulatory and respiratory systems. Severe hypoxaemia with or without hypercapnia constitutes a perfect indication for V-V ECMO configuration.

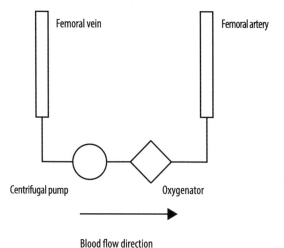

Femoral vein

Femoral artery

Centrifugal pump

Oxygenator

Blood flow direction

Figure 4. V-A ECMO configuration

Source: Author's own database.

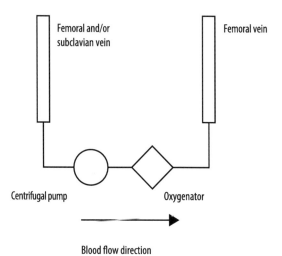

Femoral and/or
subclavian vein

Femoral vein

Centrifugal pump

Oxygenator

Blood flow direction

Figure 5. V-V ECMO configuration

Source: Author's own database.

A-V ECMO configuration is most often used in patients in cardio-respiratory failure coexistent with cardiac failure. Also severe hypothermia, poisonings, pulmonary artery embolism and cardiac arrest cases are treated with ECMO in V-A configuration. The place of catheterisation, both arterial as well as venous, may change depending on patient's condition and centre's capability. Direct catheterisation of right atrium and ascending aorta show high heamodynamic benefits. Severe forms of respiratory failure in ARDS are treated with ECMO in V-V configuration. Double-lumen catheters available on market facilitate implantation of veno-venous configuration. Experience possessed by a given centre determines the selection of transdermal or surgical method of catheterisation.

Importance of ECMO in treatment of severe hypothermia

For many years unequivocal guidelines concerning treatment of severely hypothermic patients were non-existent. Swiss Staging System of hypothermia devised in 2003, and related guidelines for treatment for patients in II, III and IV hypothermia stage devised in 2014 emphasise importance of ECMO in VA configuration in treatment of this group of patients. Obviously, this group is extremely non-homogenous as far as clinical signs are concerned. The most difficult and demanding group of the patients are those in cardiac arrest or in significant heamodynamic instability. Implementation of extracorporeal therapy in the hospital nearest the incident site or even on site of incident presents an interesting, new mode of treatment.

References

1. Gibbon J.H. *Application of a mechanical heart and lung apparatus to cardiac surgery*. Minn. Med. 1954; 37: 171–185.
2. Lim M.W. *The history of extracorporeal oxygenators*. Anaesthesia 2006; 61: 984–995.
3. Peek G., Mugford M., Tiruvoipati R. et al. *Efficacy and economic assessment of conventional ventilatory support versus extracorporeal membrane oxygenation for severe adult respiratory failure (CESAR): a multicentre randomised controlled trial*. Lancet 2009; 374: 1351–1363.

4. Davis A. et al. *Australia and New Zealand Extracorporeal membrane oxygenation (ANZ ECMO) influenza investigators.* JAMA 2009; 302: 1888–1895.
5. Schmidt M., Tachon G., Devilliers C. et al. *Blood oxygenation and decarboxylation determinants during venovenous ECMO for respiratory failure in adults.* Intens. Care Med. 2013; 39: 838–846.
6. Sidebotham D., McGeorge A., McGuinness S. et al. *Extracorporeal membrane oxygenation for treating severe cardiac and respiratory failure in adults: part 2-technical considerations.* J. Cardiothorac. Vasc. Anesth. 2010; 24: 164–172.
7. Stulak J.M., Dearani J.A., Burkhart H.M. et al. *ECMO cannulation controversies and complications.* Semin. Cardiothorac. Vasc. Anesth. 2009; 13: 176–182.
8. Kohler K., Valchanov K., Nias G. et al. *ECMO cannula review.* Perfusion 2013; 28: 114–124.
9. Toomasian J.M., Bartlett R.H. *Hemolysis and ECMO pumps in the 21st century.* Perfusion 2011; 26: 5–6.
10. Meyns B., Vercaemst L., Vandezande E. et al. *Plasma leakage of oxygenators in ECMO depends on the type of oxygenator and on patient variables.* Int. J. Artif. Organs 2005; 28: 30–34.
11. Khoshbin E., Roberts N. et al. *Polymethylpentene oxygenators have improved gas exchange capability and reduced transfusion requirements in adult extracorporeal membrane oxygenation.* ASAIO J. 2005; 51: 281–287.
12. Zafren K., Giesbrecht G.G., Danzl D.F. et al. *Wilderness Medical Society practice guidelines for the out-of-hospital evaluation and treatment of accidental hypothermia: 2014 update.* Wilderness Environ. Med. 2014; 25(4 Suppl.): 66–85.
13. Darocha T., Kosiński S., Jarosz A. et al. *Extracorporeal Rewarming From Accidental Hypothermia of Patient With Suspected Trauma.* Medicine (Baltimore) 2015; 94(27): e1086.

17

Vascular Access for Extracorporeal Circulation

Jacek Piątek, Janusz Konstanty-Kalandyk

Department of Cardiovascular Surgery and Transplantology, Jagiellonian University Collegium Medicum, Cracow, Poland
John Paul II Hospital, Cracow, Poland

Introduction

Systems of extracorporeal life support may be integrated with patient's vascular system both by central access (in the area of thorax) or a peripheral one. The basic criterion for choice of place of catheterisation is the vessel's diameter. Technological advancement has enabled reduction of catheter size with maintenance of adequate volume of blood circulating in the system. This, in turn, enables efficient support and even full substitution of circulation via peripheral access. Most often chosen catheterisation vessels are femoral vessels, less often external iliac artery, common carotid artery and subclavian artery. Apart from the diameter, anatomic topography and patient's clinical condition are further factors for choice of catheterisation place.

Femoral access

Femoral artery is a continuation of external iliac artery and the main vessel supplying blood to lower limb. Lingual ligaments divide external iliac artery from femoral artery.

The initial portion of the artery is located on frontal side of the thigh, on rear lamina of fascia lata, within femoral triangle. It is covered by superficial lamina of fascia lata and is adjacent to femoral nerve laterally and medially to femoral vein. In this location it approximates body surface, what enables the pulse palpation, whilst exerting pressure and depressing it towards illiopubic eminence makes occlusion of its lumen possible.

Surgical procedure

Patient is placed in supine position, extensive area covered with surgical drapes enables conversion to other peripheral vessels. Skin incision is usually vertical, less often horizontal or diagonal, parallel to inguinal ligament, directly above femoral artery when pulse is palpable.

In lack of presence of palpable pulse incision should be slightly medial to mid-section of inguinal ligament. Vertical incision is extended above groin, so 1/3 of the incision is above inguinal ligament and 2/3 below it. After the incision, subcutaneous tissue is exposed, fascia is incised and vascular complex is revealed – femoral artery and vein. After obtaining access to femoral artery (loop, thick suture), assessment of vessel diameter and condition of vessel wall the appropriate catheter size is chosen. The most popular artery catheter sizes are from 17 to 21 French, and venal sizes is 23 French (1 French = 0,33 mm). Femoral vein is catheterised first, then the artery. Seldinger technique is most often used. Selected vessel is punctured with a needle, then a flexible guidewire is advanced through the needle lumen. After withdrawal of the needle and widening of the puncture with a dilator, catheter is advanced over the guidewire. Then guidewire is removed and long venal catheter is placed at the entry to the right atrium, with the aid of transoesophagal echocardiography. In bad condition of femoral artery, e.g. in sclerosis, and/or risk of complications (dissection, rupture) surgical technique is used instead of Seldinger procedure, i.e. artery is incised transversally and catheter is placed directly into the vessel lumen. Additionally, in place of catheterisation vessel is sutured with monofilament, non-absorbable Prolene 5-0 suture in order to prevent bleeding on removal of catheter after termination of treatment.

After attachment and confirmation of correct functioning of ECMO system a supplementary catheter is advanced into femoral artery, distally to cannulation area, in order to improve blood circulation in the limb.

Iliac access

On account of anatomic features and more difficult surgical access – particularly in obese patients – as well as increased risk of complications this access is less frequently used.

External iliac artery bifurcates off common iliac artery and is its medio--lateral final branch. Bifurcation of common iliac artery is located at the level of lower border of L5 vertebra and somewhat medially from lumbosacral joint line, i.e. about 4 cm laterally from the medial line. The artery is directed anteriorly, inferiorly and laterally, forming an arch with its concavity medially and down. Its direct continuation, in lower limb, is femoral artery.

In the elderly the artery can be meandering.

Incision is made about 2 cm about inguinal ligament, whose line is formed by anterior superior iliac spine and pubic symphisis. After severance of fascia and parting of transverse muscles iliac artery is exposed and catheterised using similar technique as in femoral artery.

Subclavian access

Right and left subclavian arteries originate differently. Right subclavian artery comes off brachiocephalic trunk at the root of the neck, left subclavian artery is one of three branches of aorta in superior mediastinum. Subclavian artery may be divided into three parts: ascending, apical, and descending. After it arises off, subclavian artery lies adjacent to pleural cupula – together with brachial plexus it passes through scalene muscles, through posterior gap in scalene muscles next to the first rib. In the next section subclavian artery passes to supraclavicular fossa, where it is located superficially, almost subcutaneously. The vessel terminates on anterior border of the first rib, below the clavicle where it continues as axillary artery. In rare instances right subclavian artery comes off as additional, fourth, leftmost branch of aorta (located in vicinity of transition of aortic arch into descending aorta). This is termed aberrant right subclavian artery (*arteria lusoria*).

Two options of artery access exist: above and below the clavicle. On account of topography and resulting risk of complications as well as – crucially – small diameter of the vessel rendering direct placement of arterial catheter impossible, this method is seldom used. Often, the access is possible only by use of artificial vascular graft (end to side technique) and advancement of catheter into the graft.

Carotid access

Common carotid artery is the main arterial vessel supplying head and neck with blood. Left carotid artery comes off aortic arch, and right one from brachiocephalic trunk. Within neck, it runs adjacent to internal jugular vein and vagus nerve inside carotid sheath. Within carotid triangle, it emerges from under anterior border of sternocleidomastoid, making easy pulse palpation possible. In its upper run it forms carotid sinus. Common carotid artery bifurcates at the level of C3–C4 into internal and external carotid arteries. Within neck, common carotid artery gives off no branches prior to bifurcation.

After preparation of operating field and rotation of head in the opposite direction a skin incision is made along the line connecting earlobe and suprasternal notch. After lateral repositioning of sternocleidomastoid head and severance of fascia, common carotid artery is visualised.

The diameter of carotid artery – similarly as of subclavian artery – renders direct access practically impossible. Catheterisation is possible only with vascular graft. For this reason, this access technique is not in standard use, but practiced only in extraordinary circumstances.

Recommendations for emergency care

Implementation of ECMO may constitute the only chance for survival for severely hypothermic patients. In majority of patients in hypothermia who are admitted to cardiac surgery centres severe circulatory failure or cardiac arrest are witnessed. Vascular access is thus challenging and time for the procedure is limited. For these reasons the above described catheterisation areas should be particularly protected from the very beginning of rescue procedures. It happens, that during the rescue multiple vascular access attempts are made, for instance so as to obtain blood samples. Each vessel puncture of this kind may, in coexistent coagulopathy, cause vessel damage, haemorrhage and alteration of anatomical topography, and, as a consequence, impede or render impossible obtaining of a "lifeline." Major vessels damage during rescue endeavours should be avoided at all costs, particularly of the femoral vessels. It is crucial to avoid both vessel punctures as well as injuries to groin area (e.g. with heat sources used for external rewarming). In case of unequivocal necessity to obtain vascular access in the critical areas, real-time ultrasonography and selection of experienced personnel is recommended.

18

Problems and Pitfalls of Qualification for Extracorporeal Treatment of Patients in Severe Hypothermia

Anna Jarosz[1,2], Sylweriusz Kosiński[2,3,4], Tomasz Darocha[1,2], Hubert Hymczak[1,2], Peter Paal[5], Rafał Drwiła[1,2]

[1] Severe Hypothermia Treatment Centre, Department of Anaesthesiology and Intensive Care, John Paul II Hospital, Cracow, Poland
[2] "Heat for Life" Foundation, Cracow, Poland
[3] Department of Anesthesiology and Intensive Care, Pulmonary Hospital, Zakopane, Poland
[4] Tatra Mountain Rescue Service, Zakopane, Poland
[5] Department of Anaesthesiology and Critical Care Medicine, University Hospital Innsbruck, Austria; and Barts Heart Centre, St Bartholomew's Hospital, Barts Health NHS Trust, Queen Mary University of London, United Kingdom; International Commission for Mountain Emergency Medicine (ICAR MEDCOM)

If indications for extracorporeal rewarming in hypothermia are clearly defined, the problems one might encounter in practice have not been, as yet, delineated. Isolated reports on "qualification pitfalls" appear in certain case studies, but majority of these constitute only relative contraindications. In patients with instability of cardiovascular system, and cardiac arrest in particular, decision to qualify for extracorporeal rewarming must be immediate. At the same time, diagnostic possibilities are significantly limited (incoming reports from emergency medical teams or mountain rescue services, patients undergoing resuscitation or extremely unstable). In such instances not qualification, but denial of extracorporeal treatment may present the greatest challenge on both clinical as well as ethical planes.

The compilation of problems and pitfalls experienced during qualification procedure is based upon several months of work of Severe Hypothermia Treatment Centre coordinators in Kraków. It is until now the only centre specialising in extracorporeal rewarming in Poland, and the only one operating according to proprietary, uniform algorithm. This has allowed to observe recurrence of certain conditions, assess their importance and draw appropriate conclusions. ECMO therapy carries a risk of grave complications, but majority of these can be avoided by means of proper qualification procedure and avoidance of factors which affect the very treatment. As emphasised before, the problems described below constitute merely relative contraindications, and thanks to good long term outcomes of extracorporeal rewarming, they should be considered in relation to a complete disorder evaluation and discussed by the team involved in the treatment.

Thrombocytopenia and/or clinically important anaemia

These disorders are present in patients belonging to so called "underclass", but also in the elderly, neglected and malnutrition stricken victims of "urban hypothermia." The values of haemoglobin seen in our patients reached even 3.6 mg/dL and thrombocyte count 18,000/mL. It should be stressed that even such low parameters do not constitute a contraindication for extracorporeal rewarming, yet require intervention. The most important challenge in such cases is establishing absence of haemorrhage.

Proposed procedure:

- establishing absence of haemorrhage (clinical examination, USG, CT);
- medical history, diagnostic aimed at hepatic or renal insufficiencies, neoplastic diseases (terminal phase);
- packed red blood cells and/or platelet concentrate transfusion – target values of haemoglobin: 9–10 mg/dL, platelets: 50,000/mL minimum.

Peritoneal cavity free fluid of unknown origin

It may be occasionally observed, usually in the elderly, as a consequence of hypothermia or chronic disorders. Typically it is diagnosed during routine USG examination performed in order to determine trauma presence. The condition, if not a sign of fresh post-traumatic haemorrhage, does not constitute contraindication for extracorporeal rewarming.
Proposed procedure:

- establishing absence of haemorrhage (clinical examination, USG, CT);
- medical history, diagnostic aimed at hepatic or renal insufficiencies, neoplastic diseases (terminal phase).

Head injury/intracranial haemorrhage of unknown onset

Detailed medical history and image diagnostics undertaken in order to determine absence of trauma are essential steps to be taken in qualifying patient to extracorporeal rewarming. Systemic anticoagulation therapy may precipitate fatal haemorrhage even in insignificant injuries, particularly in closed body compartments (e.g. cranial cavity). Even though in some few centres ECMO is implemented in patients after polytrauma, such therapy necessitates use of special drainage system and material experience in such treatment [1, 2]. Abnormalities in intracranial space need not signify recent trauma, but each such abnormality should be reviewed by an experienced neurosurgeon.
Proposed procedure:

- neurosurgical consultation (indications for craniotomy?, risk of bleeding after heparinisation?);
- extended coagulation system laboratory tests (including thromboelastometry if available);
- qualification for extracorporeal rewarming after written opinion by neurosurgeon.

Age limits

Age of patient does not comprise an issue for implementation of rewarming with ECMO. The youngest of the patients we had treated was 2 years old, the oldest – 83. In both patients full recovery ensued. Availability of extracorporeal therapy in younger patients may, however, be a problem. Adults-oriented cardiac surgery centres usually do not possess equipment and experience in treating children.

Proposed procedure:

- prior development of cooperation measures with children cardiac surgery centres (or any other ones possessing suitable equipment and trained staff);
- establishing forms and principles for patient transport.

Bleeding from external auditory canal

It may occur in patients in whom ear canal temperature measurement was attempted in prehospital or early in-hospital phase. Lack of experience in epitympanic probe placement may cause rupture of the eardrum. If no head or intracranial injury occurs, an isolated tympanic membrane or external auditory canal tissue damage do not constitute a contraindication for ECMO therapy.

Proposed procedure:

- otoscopy, in case of doubts: otolaryngological consultation, CT of the head;
- establishing absence of cranium fracture or intracranial haemorrhage.

Use of infrared detection thermometers (IRED)

Use of popular IRED thermometers – particularly in prehospital phase – may disturb the entire procedure. As mentioned before (see Chapter 4), one of the goals in hypothermia treatment is measurement of core temperature. Methods based on infrared radiation intensity are inaccurate in hypothermia to such a degree that they should not be be used [3, 4]. In cold ambient temperature tympanic membrane temperature measured with infrared method is lower by 1.4°C on average from core temperature. The result of the measurement, moreover, depends on the technique used (up to 51% of the measurements do not reflect core temperature). The influence of environment temperature, neighbouring tissues, as well as water and snow which may penetrate into auditory canal, is also significant. If medical history implies that measurement was done with IRED thermometer, prior to decision to initiate extracorporeal rewarming verification of actual core temperature with recommended means should be attempted at any cost.

Proposed procedure:

- obligatory verification of place and technique of temperature measurement implemented by emergency teams;
- clinical examination (neurological condition, circulatory system condition, ECG);
- verification of IRED measurement (exception: cardiac arrest on arrival of emergency team or during initial phase of care).

Iatrogenic injury of femoral blood vessels

This is usually caused by attempts of cannulation of arterial vein/artery during emergency care in emergency department (particularly in hypotensive or cardiac arrest patients). In coexistent coagulopathy haemorrhage to retroperitoneal space may occur. Catheters necessary for extracorporeal blood circulation are introduced also via femoral vessels. Their injury may rule out or significantly hinder catheter placement, and as a consequence rule out extracorporeal rewarming.

Proposed procedure:

- information from emergency department to emergency team on site of incident about the vascular access necessary for ECMO and possible consequences of haemorrhage;
- rule of not puncturing femoral vessels (at least unilaterally);
- if puncture/cannulation deemed indispensable, use of USG visualisation is recommended.

Poisonings

Among patients undergoing consultation with SHTC coordinator via telephone one case of carbon monoxide and one of isopropyl alcohol poisoning, and a few cases of alcohol intoxication were reported. The poisonings are on one hand a possible primary cause of hypothermia, on the other may pose a problem in differentiation of causes for loss of consciousness and clinical evaluation of hypothermia (particularly in prehospital phase).
Proposed procedure:

- testing for ethanol and other toxins depending on medical history and clinical examination result (e.g. severe acidosis not corresponding with hypothermia stage);
- treatment of causes (e.g. hyperbaric oxygen therapy) before commencement of rewarming (exception: patients in cardiac arrest);
- alcohol intoxication does not comprise a problem during extracorporeal rewarming.

Hypoglycaemia

It is a relatively frequent phenomenon (about 25% of the patients), usually witnessed in chronic hypothermia (urban hypothermia or hypothermia associated with physical fatigue). This problem is important for prognosis, as hypoglycaemia is one of primary causes of hypothermia (risk of neuroglycopenia before cooling). Hypoglycaemia may have its onset also during rewarming as a consequence of metabolic rate acceleration, restoring of insulin activity and increase in glucose utilisation.

Proposed procedure:

- obligatory, as early as possible glucose level test in all hypothermic patients;
- constant glucose supplementation in chronic hypothermia;
- regular glucose testing, also during extracorporeal rewarming.

Haemodynamically stable patient with Tc ≤ 28°C

Literature and our experience prove that clinical signs of hypothermia (neurological condition, cardiovascular system condition) do not always correspond to core temperature. This is often caused by error in measurement, but not always. Adaptation capabilities of human organism are beyond measure. Both medical as well as popular press bring descriptions of people who managed to perform often complicated tasks in challenging conditions and in severe hypothermia. Among patients treated in SHTC in three patients in borderline circulatory stability cardiac arrest occurred in initial phase of treatment. Therefore one should not show negligence to incoming information where clinical condition of the patient fails to reflect temperature measured. Unfortunately, no objective factor which could indicate increased probability of cardiac arrest in hypothermic patients has been identified. Thus, especially in initial phase of treatment, particular caution should be maintained, as the changes in patient's overall condition can be rapid. It is worth emphasising that the problem described here is not rare and can affect up to 25% of the patients.

Proposed procedure:

- ensuring of possibility of ECMO treatment during non-invasive rewarming.

Increased level of creatine kinase (CK) and creatine kinase isoenzyme MB (CK-MB)

This problem occurs often and was observed in 70% of patients treated by SHTC. Increased activity of CK-MB may raise suspicion of acute coronary syndrome (particularly in combination with ECG abnormalities) and delay diagnosis of hypothermia. Usually, however, increased levels of CK and CK-MB result from intense muscle activity accompanying hypothermia (shivering) and do not require specific treatment. Very high levels of CK (in one of our patients 87 191 U) may indicate rhabdomyolysis, resulting from e.g. frostbites or compartment syndrome, and require further diagnostics.

Proposed procedure:

- elevated CK, CK-MB do not comprise a contraindication for extracorporeal rewarming;
- if clinical signs of compartment syndrome are present, surgical intervention (fasciotomy) should be considered.

Summary

Qualifying patient for extracorporeal rewarming is not an easy task, even if fixed criteria and procedure exist. On account of necessity for at least partial heparinisation, the primary task is detection of active bleeding. In presence of signs of shock, anaemia, thrombocytopenia, and in ambiguous image diagnostics results, differentiation between hypothermia-induced and hypovolemic shock accompanied by hypothermia is very difficult. This and other qualification pitfalls prove that it is fairly easy to find indications for extracorporeal rewarming, yet it is problematic to critically asses contraindications for such a treatment.

References

1. Arlt M., Philipp A., Voelkel S. et al. *Extracorporeal membrane oxygenation in severe trauma patients with bleeding shock*. Resuscitation 2010; 81: 804–809.
2. Biderman P., Einav S., Fainblu M. et al. *Extracorporeal life support in patients with multiple injuries and severe respiratory failure: A single-center experience*. J. Trauma Acute Care Surg. 2013; 75: 907–912.
3. Rogers I.R., O'Brien D.L., Wee C. et al. *Infrared emission tympanic thermometers cannot be relied upon in a wilderness setting*. Wilderness Environ. Med. 1999; 10: 201–203.
4. Bagey J., Judelson D.A., Spiering B.A. et al. *Validity of field expedient devices to assess core temperature during exercise in the cold*. Aviat. Space Environ. Med. 2011; 82: 1098–1103.

19

Procedure of Extracorporeal Treatment of Hypothermic Patients

Tomasz Darocha[1,2], Sylweriusz Kosiński[2,3,4], Anna Jarosz[1,2], Hubert Hymczak[1,2], Robert Gałązkowski[5], Tomasz Sanak[2,6,7], Jerzy Sadowski[8], Bogusław Kapelak[8], Rafał Drwiła[1,2]

[1] Severe Hypothermia Treatment Centre, Department of Anaesthesiology and Intensive Care, John Paul II Hospital, Chair of Anaesthesiology and Intensive Care, Jagiellonian University Collegium Medicum, Cracow, Poland
[2] "Heat for Life" Foundation, Cracow, Poland
[3] Department of Anaesthesiology and Intensive Care, Pulmonary Hospital, Zakopane, Poland
[4] Tatra Mountain Rescue Service, Zakopane, Poland
[5] Department of Emergency Medical Services, Medical University, Helicopter Emergency Medical Service, Warsaw, Poland
[6] Department of Disaster Medicine and Emergency Care, Chair of Anaesthesiology and Intensive Care, Jagiellonian University Collegium Medicum, Cracow, Poland
[7] Department of Battlefield Medicine, Military Institute of Medicine, Warsaw, Poland
[8] The Department of Cardiovascular Surgery and Transplantation, Jagiellonian University Collegium Medicum, John Paul II Hospital, Cracow, Poland

In June 2013 the first Polish system of qualification for extracorporeal rewarming of patients in severe hypothermia was developed, it encompasses with its reach the patients of Lesser Poland Voivodeship. The core of the system is Severe Hypothermia Treatment Centre (SHTC) by Department of Anaesthesiology and Intensive Care at John Paul II Hospital in Kraków. Its objective is treatment of severe stages of hypothermia with extracorporeal membrane oxygenation (ECMO) method as well support of cooperating entities with knowledge and aiding them in decision making process. The concept of the entire programme and procedure itself were based upon experts' recommendations as well as experience of other centres in the world [1–3], but reach and range of activity of SHTC are exceptional.

The idea of the system development was based on previous experience of the systems originators and information gathered via countrywide questionnaire concerning hypothermia diagnosis and treatment [4]. Hypothermia, and its severe stages in particular, is diagnosed sporadically, but its incidence rate is probably higher than implied by the official statistical data. The means of treatment which were put to use have not always been successful, and instances of extracorporeal techniques were merely anecdotal. We assumed that the only way of increasing the efficacy of treatment is developing a system which will provide full care of the patients – from early identification, through safe transportation, up to present-day and efficient possibilities of rewarming and life support. Initially the victims of acute exposure hypothermia (e.g. in the mountains, after cold water immersion) were in the scope of our interest, but, according to our expectations, chronic urban hypothermia has proven to be the greatest challenge.

The system would fail to function without broad educational and information campaign. Series of trainings for physicians, nurses, paramedics and also for the police, fire departments, and other entities cooperating with the system was initiated. During the meetings the means of recognising and treatment of hypothermia were discussed, population at risk was identified, and newly developed algorithm was presented. Educational materials and information on methods of notifying system coordinator reached all emergency departments (20 emergency departments proper and 11 inpatient departments), ambulance stations, fire departments, railroad police units, employees of 6 national parks, border guard, and police departments within the voivodeship. Agreement of cooperation was signed with mountain rescue services (all groups of Polish Mountain Rescue Service as well as Tatra Mountain Rescue Service). Upon the agreement the rescuers are obliged to report all search and rescue missions conducted on their respective areas of operation occurring between 1 October and 1 April. Thanks to this, system coordinators have a capacity of early initiation of response and coordination of preparation steps for implementation of extracorporeal rewarming.

Establishing a role of coordinator available 24 hours a day via telephone was crucial for the system's success. The tasks of coordinator include consultation of hypothermia cases diagnosed on the territory of the voivodeship, competent aid during diagnostics and treatment in medical centres, as well as potential qualification for extracorporeal rewarming. The coordinators work as volunteers, the team currently comprises five people. Incoming calls are automatically registered with form devised for this purpose. It happens that coordination of rescue efforts of one patient lasts for several hours and necessitates several dozens (!) of phone calls. In a few instances cooperation and simultaneous work of two coordinators was indispensable. Apart from the above mentioned tasks coordinators carry on educational work, perform periodic analyses of efficacy of the therapy and – what is vital – they pass on observations and informations about treatment outcomes to cooperating entities and participants of rescue efforts. It was realised that even a succinct feedback ameliorates system's integrity, improves information exchange and facilitates organisation of future operations. In order to improve effectiveness of coordination we have started a database of cardiac surgery departments in neighbouring voivodeships, emergency medical teams bases, as well as availability of monitoring equipment and – importantly – automated chest compressions devices. This enables quick availability of devices which may be indispensable on site of incident and during transportation. All, even sudden shortages were catered for thanks to close and effective cooperation with Dispatch Centre in Kraków and Medical Air Rescue.

All entities responsible for all 115 state land ambulances on the territory of the voivodeship were notified about the operation and system principles. Information about diagnosis and treatment of hypothermia were uploaded into portable computers comprising the ambulance equipment.

Five HEMS helicopters operating in the area were equipped with specialised low-reading thermometers, and the personnel was prepared for transportation of hypothermic patients. Steps were taken to replace shortages in equipment and make sure that all measuring devices are uniform in all cooperating entities so as to enable measurements of low body temperature of the patients already in the initial phase of treatment. It should be stated here that we continue works on development of a new portable and accurate thermometer for emergency care units.

Efforts were made to establish formal standards concerning treatment of hypothermia. Lesser Poland Voivodeship's consultant in the field of emergency medicine has issued an official recommendation for emergency departments and inpatient departments:

"Within rescue procedures in unconscious patients whose medical history may indicate hypothermia core temperature measurement is obligatory. In case of detection of core temperature below 28°C a telephone consultation with extracorporeal treatment of severe hypothermia coordinator is recommended."

A recommendation for emergency care team personnel was also published:

"Within rescue procedures in unconscious patients in whom medical history may indicate hypothermia temperature measurement is obligatory. In case of detection of temperature below 30°C a telephone consultation with extracorporeal treatment of severe hypothermia coordinator of Lesser Poland Voivodeship is recommended." (Both documents are available [in Polish] at: www.hipotermia.edu.pl).

SHTC in Kraków is the only centre in Poland currently cooperating with International Hypothermia Registry in Geneva, Switzerland, and sharing often precious information for purposes of statistical analyses and scientific research.

Qualifying criteria for extracorporeal rewarming at SHTC are as follows:

• stage III of hypothermia according to Swiss Staging System, with clinically present circulatory instability;
• cardiac arrest in course of hypothermia – stage IV, on condition of continuation of resuscitation throughout the entire transportation process (mechanical chest compressions systems are recommended);
• verification of hypothermia with core temperature measurement (oesophagus, rectum, urinary bladder, tympanic membrane;
• core temperature < 28°C;
• negative V hypothermia stage (signs of irreversible death);
• in patients with bodily injury or suspicion of disorders in which administration of heparin is contraindicated – conducting of image diagnostics (CT in trauma scan mode).

It is worth noting that we do not always manage to ensure observation of all necessary criteria. The primary problem is technical side of temperature measurement. It happens that time-consuming theoretical explanation and "live" counselling via telephone during measurement procedure prove necessary. In many cases we mindfully refrained from enforcing certain criteria on account of persuasive clinical picture, as we aim to resolve all doubts with the greatest good of the patient in mind.

We have assigned the following tasks to the Emergency Medical Teams and Medical Air Rescue:

- clinical assessment, assessment according to Swiss Staging System, trauma examination, measurement of temperature with available equipment;
- in case of severe hypothermia suspicion (stage III with signs of circulatory instability and stage IV according to Swiss Staging System) – notification of medical dispatcher or regional consultants in the field of emergency medicine;
- transportation to destination treatment centre;
- if necessary – commencement of cardio-pulmonary resuscitation and its continuation throughout the transportation process.

It might appear that the tasks listed above are mere basics. In reality, however, medical emergency teams are burdened with the most challenging duties: diagnostic sensitivity, collection of complete medical history, prevention of complications which may occur in the early phase of treatment, sometimes challenging secondary transportation process to SHTC. These duties demand both knowledge and experience, which are possessed and quickly acquired by our colleagues in ambulances and helicopters.

Finally, we would like to present roles and tasks of emergency departments and intensive care units personnel:

- medical examination performed by physician, measurement/verification of core temperature;
- telephone consultation with medical centre possessing extracorporeal rewarming (ECMO, extracorporeal life support) capability;
- ensuring CT in trauma scan mode in case of injury or suspected injury;
- determining presence or absence of disorders in which heparin administration is contraindicated – provision of necessary diagnostic measures;
- continuation of resuscitation combined with rewarming with available non-invasive methods;
- organisation of transportation of the patient to medical centre with extracorporeal treatment capability.

What is important – we assumed that the final decision to commence rewarming procedure with extracorporeal method is made by medical personnel of the centre where the treatment is to be conducted (i.e. in our case by SHTC staff). As we always keep in mind the greatest good of the patient in mind, it happens that on the basis of acquired information we make a decision to continue treatment in our centre . Extracorporeal rewarming and support are an invasive method (see Chapter 14) which is associated with – occasionally significant – risk. Both coordinator as well as SHTC staff have to make an informed choice, which is not always compliant with local centre's personnel preference. Possessing increasingly larger knowledge and experience with with every new patient, we are able to avoid growing number of pitfalls of qualification and treatment [5].

Present experience

Until 20 Janurary 2016, 25 patients were treated in SHTC. In all, severe stages of hypothermia were diagnosed (core temperature below 28°C) and all met pre-established qualification criteria. 13 patients experienced cardiac arrest and were admitted during ongoing resuscitation (cardiac arrest duration until implementation of extracorporeal rewarming was from 107 to 345 minutes). In the remaining 12 patients spontaneous circulation was present, but on admission the patients were unconscious and in cardiogenic shock. In each of these groups 5 deaths occurred (jointly 10 deaths, overall inhospital fatality was 40%). It is worth noting that in all patients treated, normothermia was achieved, and causes of death were complications resulting from accompanying disorders. The remaining patients (15) were discharged in overall good condition, without neurological deficits (GCS 15, CPC 1).

References

1. Brown D.J., Brugger H., Boyd J. et al. *Accidental hypothermia*. N. Engl. J. Med. 2012; 367: 1930–1938.
2. Durrer B., Brugger H., Syme D. et al. *The medical on-site treatment of hypothermia ICAR-MEDCOM recommendation*. High Alt. Med. Biol. 2003; 4: 99–10.
3. Soar J., Perkins G.D., Abbas G. et al. *European Resuscitation Council Guidelines for Resuscitation 2010 Section 8. Cardiac arrest in special circumstances: Electrolyte abnormalities, poisoning, drowning, accidental hypothermia, hyperthermia, asthma, anaphylaxis, cardiac surgery, trauma, pregnancy, electrocution.* Resuscitation 2010; 81: 1400–1433.
4. Kosiński S., Darocha T., Gałązkowski R. et al. *Accidental hypothermia in Poland – estimation of prevalence, diagnostic methods and treatment*. Scand. J. Trauma Resusc. Emerg. Med. 2015; 23: 13.
5. Jarosz A., Kosiński S., Darocha T. et al. *The problems and pitfalls of qualification for extracorporeal rewarming in severe accidental hypothermia. A preliminary report from the Severe Hypothermia Treatment Centre.* Kraków (in press).

20

Recommendation of National Consultant in the Field on Emergency Medicine

RECOMMENDATION FOR EMERGENCY DEPARTMENTS/INPATIENT DE-PARTMENTS PERSONNEL CONCERNING MANAGEMENT OF HYPOTHER-MIC PATIENTS.

Within rescue procedures in unconscious patients whose medical history may indicate hypothermia core temperature measurement is obligatory. In case of detection of core temperature below 28°C a telephone consultation with physician on duty at the nearest Anaesthesiology and Intensive Care Unit in a hospital with cardiac surgery department, and thus possibility of implementation of extracorporeal rewarming with extracorporeal circulation system (CPB) or ECMO, is recommended.

Prof. Jerzy Robert Ładny, MD, PhD
National Consultant in the Field on Emergency Medicine

21

Accidental Hypothermia: the Need for the International Hypothermia Registry

Beat H. Walpoth[1], Marie Meyer[2], Christophe Gaudet-Blavignac[3], Philippe Baumann[3], Pierre Gilquin[3], Christian Lovis[3]

[1] Division of Cardiovascular Surgery, University Hospitals of Geneva, Switzerland
[2] Dept. of Anesthesia, University Hospital, Lausanne, Switzerland
[3] Division of Medical Information Sciences, University Hospitals of Geneva, Switzerland

Accidental hypothermia can be of multiple aetiologies and is often related to an accident in a cold environment and contrasts with urban hypothermia. People living in the cold such as workers, fishermen and military personnel are at risk. More recently there is an increase in unprepared lay people practicing leisure activities such as winter sports, thus exposing themselves to hypothermia in case of an accident. Most of the cases concern mild hypothermia which does not need hospitalization or medical assistance. In contrast, deep hypothermia, with or without cardiac arrest, is rare and carries a high mortality in healthy adults and children [1, 2, 3].

Induced hypothermia which has been used for cardiac surgery as well as therapeutic hypothermia used for brain ischaemia, are medically indicated and highly monitored and therefore cannot be compared to accidental hypothermia. Patients with induced hypothermia may reach the same degree (< 28°C) but are in controlled narcosis and are normally cooled down and rewarmed by Cardiopulmonary Bypass (CPB) [4]. Therapeutic hypothermia cools the patient to mild hypothermia (32–34°C) to enhance a better and faster functional brain recovery [5].

The concept of applying the technique of CPB rewarming, as used in induced deep hypothermic cardiac arrest, to victims of accidental hypothermia with temperatures below 28°C and cardio-respiratory arrest was initiated successfully by Prof. Ueli Althaus at the University Hospital Insel in Bern, Switzerland over 30 years ago [6]. Since that time our team and other Swiss universities started to use this method and we published a multi-centre study showing a long-term sequelae-free survival rate of 47% after rewarming of 32 deep accidental hypothermic patients in cardiac arrest using cardiopulmonary bypass (CPB) [7]. Due to the fact that many patients died from post-rewarming complications, we and others have shown the beneficial effect of using extra-corporeal life support (ECLS) such as prolonged ECMO use after rewarming for cardiovascular and pulmonary dysfunctions [8, 9].

Accidental hypothermia requiring medical assistance is fortunately relatively rare and therefore there is a lack of evidence for issuing recommendations based on solid statistics. Case reports with positive outcomes are often published, whereas the negative outcome patients are not described but much could be learned from the latter [10, 11]. The rewarming and management of moderate or deep hypothermic victims (body temperature < 32°C) remains a real challenge for medical and scientific teams. Additionally, no good outcome predictors exist except for potassium which would facilitate the triage and decision-making of the adequate best treatment for such victims.

The International Hypothermia Registry (IHR) was created in Geneva five years ago in order to gather a large number of accidental hypothermia cases. It includes all cases of accidental hypothermia with a body temperature < 32°C, regardless of aetiology and outcome.

Access rights for the IHR can be obtained by completing a form. There are 4 levels of access rights: Case editor, Centre reviewer, Centre supervisor, Registry supervisor. It is the responsibility of each participating centre to obtain ethical approval for entering their patients and informed consent is advisable. Outcome being the main endpoint of the Registry, it is hoped that the treating doctor contacts the patient one year after the accident in order to complete the outcome section. The IHR is composed of three main sections: the pre-hospital data (accident features and medical features); the hospital data (pre-rewarming data, rewarming techniques and post rewarming ICU and hospital follow-up) and a one-year outcome (follow up of complications and quality of life). The International Hypothermia Registry (IHR) is web-based. The registry is hosted on the